STOLEN *Youth*

MY DAUGHTER'S BATTLE WITH KIDNEY DISEASE

John C. Bishop and Kristen M. Bishop
with Sean Johannesen

Stolen Youth
Copyright © 2021 by John C. Bishop and
Kristen M. Bishop with Sean Johannesen

All rights reserved. No part of this publication may be reproduced, distributed, or transmitted in any form or by any means, including photocopying, recording, or other electronic or mechanical methods, without the prior written permission of the author, except in the case of brief quotations embodied in critical reviews and certain other non-commercial uses permitted by copyright law.

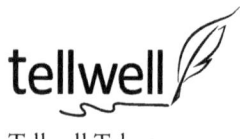

Tellwell Talent
www.tellwell.ca

ISBN
978-0-2288-6655-8 (Paperback)
978-0-2288-6656-5 (eBook)

Table of Contents

Acknowledgments vii
A Note to the Reader ix
An Additional Note to our American Readers xi

Part 1: Early Warnings

    The Call 3
    Remarkably Ordinary 6
    Spring Break 10
    Heart Tests 13
    Pediatrician Appointment 16
    Blood Work 18
    Blood Test Results 20
    Meeting Dr. Crocker 22

Part 2: Fight for Survival

    Surviving 27
    Settling In 29
    The Biopsy 31
    Dialysis Catheter 33
    Biopsy Results, Dialysis Begins 37
    Meeting Dr. Acott 40
    Day of Rest 42
    Meeting the Transplant Nurse 43
    Nose Tube 47
    Searching for a Donor 49
    Dialysis Stopped 51
    On the Up-and-Up 54
    Blessed Boredom 55
    Another Day in 'Paradise' 57
    Grace under Pressure 59
    Thrown from the Train 60

Part 3: If at First You Don't Succeed...

Support System 65
The Diet Police 67
A Hat Trick of Good Days 70
Mother's Day 73
The Ward 75
Bitter Medicine 76
Mooseheads! 79
School Days 81
"One in Twenty" 83
In Isolation 84
In Training 87
Wake-Up Call 89
Home Away from Home 91
Some Sad News; Another Crisis 93
The Award Goes To… 95
Special Delivery 97
Another Man Down 98
Back to Square One 99

Part 4: Try Again!

Thinking Positive 103
Second Chance 105
Silent Alarms 107
Finally Home 109
Timing 111
Fountain of Generosity 113
Meeting the Shrink 116
Raleigh and Back 118

Part 5: The Big Day

Final Tests 123
Kristen Checks In 125
John Checks In 127
The Big Day 129

The Day After.. 134
Simulect, Take Two 136
In Recovery.. 138
Stents, Staples, and the Great Outdoors 141
Third Time Lucky?... 144

Part 6: Different Lives

Checked Out! 147
Post-op Biopsies 149
Back to School 151
University 153
A New Journey 157
John: The Fear Never Leaves... 158
Kristen: Looking Forward 160

Afterword..163

Acknowledgments

Although I've wanted to write this story for a long time, having majored in Business at university, I wasn't exactly equipped with the right set of tools to turn our story into a finished book. Enter Sean Johannesen. Sean is someone I met through volunteer work at my church. I had no idea at the time how gifted he was. We began to talk, and almost immediately he volunteered to help with the project. There is no doubt in my mind that this book would not have made it this far without his help, so we will be eternally grateful to him.

Some other wonderful people were instrumental in making this book a reality. Janet Sketchley provided invaluable expertise and guidance, bringing both her experience as a published author and her excellent suggestions as a beta reader (and on top of that, helping us come up with the perfect title!). Debbie Bishop graciously read through the finished manuscript and allowed us to include her in pictures in the final book. Our daughters, Danielle and Allison, and their friends Megan and Katie Beger of Michigan, also allowed us to include them in some of the photographs—thanks so much, girls! We're also extremely grateful to Karen Baer and author Sara B. Gauldin, who both took the time to read the final manuscript and offer constructive feedback and encouragement.

The people at Disney kindly gave us permission to show their beloved character Minnie Mouse in one of the images, and the Montréal Canadiens Hockey Club generously allowed us to use both a photograph of one of their star players and a letter from then-president Pierre Boivin in the book. These images were helpful to the story, and we're very grateful to both organizations for giving us permission to use them.

Of course, the book wouldn't have happened at all if it weren't for the support that we received from so many people during that difficult year when Kristen was in and out of the hospital. First and foremost, I would like to thank the incredible staff at the IWK hospital. Dr. Crocker (who has now passed on) and Dr. Acott were there for us at every step, explaining the process so that a layman like myself could understand it. These two doctors were known around the world for their tireless work in the field of nephrology, and we knew we were extremely fortunate to have them leading Kristen's surgical team.

I cannot say enough about the wonderful nurses and support staff at the 6 North clinic of the IWK. They made us feel like part of their extended family during our six-month ordeal, always showing compassion and care when times got rough, and seeming to know exactly what to do in any situation that arose. I can only offer a great big hug and thanks for everything they did for our family.

Many of our friends and family members pulled us through a very difficult time. They put smiles on our faces when they were needed and sent Kristen thoughtful cards, and even occasional gifts, to show us how much they cared for us and for a successful outcome. Some, like John and Maureen Sullivan, went above and beyond the call of duty, providing us with help in so many ways that we could never possibly repay them.

When my mother was alive, she knew Catholic nuns who were stationed all over the globe. She tapped into this resource, and we had prayers coming in from everywhere. In addition to that, our church community also supported us with prayers. As I've said many times, I believe it was because of these people's prayers that we had such a successful outcome. I will be forever in their debt.

Finally, I would like to thank my daughter Kristen for being so strong and centred throughout this ordeal. I learned a great deal from her positive attitude. Even when her daily medical trials seemed impossible to bear, Kristen fought through it all like a trouper, displaying incredible perseverance and determination. These qualities have also served her well in the years since, and she's been an inspiration to me time after time.

—John C. Bishop, March 2020

A Note to the Reader

Although memoirs are often written from the viewpoint of a single author, this one benefits from the combined memories of two people. Most of the story comes from John Bishop's point of view, as he describes how he nearly lost his daughter Kristen to kidney failure. Kristen's accounts of that time appear throughout the book, and I've formatted them so that you can easily tell them apart.

As you read, you'll notice how Kristen's memories complement those of her father, and how together, they create a compelling picture of that difficult time—no mean feat, given that they were recalling details from about fifteen years earlier.

Occasionally, though, you'll notice that their memories contradict each other—sometimes humorously, other times poignantly. If you're a student of human nature and the vagaries of memory, then I think you'll find these differences fascinating.

I have enjoyed working on this project, with all its complements and contradictions, and I am grateful to John and Kristen for being so open and candid in recounting all that they went through. I hope that your experience of reading their story will be just as enjoyable and enlightening.

—Sean Johannesen, March 2020

An Additional Note to our American Readers

If you've never visited Canada, then before continuing, you may find it useful to read the following.

First, as you read our story, you'll probably notice that some words appear to be misspelled. As with many parts of our eclectic culture, the Canadian language borrows from both British and American conventions. Canadians don't really notice, but other readers may be left scratching their heads at our odd mix of American and British spellings.

True to our Canadian roots, we offer our sincerest apologies for any confusion this may cause.

The second thing you'll probably notice is that we don't mention anywhere in the book how Kristen's extensive, six-month treatment was paid for. Considering how serious her condition was and how long she was in the hospital, it may seem odd that we never mention having worried about whether our insurance would cover everything, or whether we had to exhaust our savings or sell our house to pay for her treatment.

This will make sense if you're familiar with the Canadian health care system.

Canada uses a health insurance program that is actually built on 13 separate health plans, one for each province and territory. Each plan operates under the umbrella of the federal government's Health Care Act.

Reading the Act is about as exciting as you could expect any government document to be, but its basic goal is very clear: to ensure that every Canadian has "reasonable access to health services without financial or other barriers."

Unlike the U.K. government (which directly employs about a million people and runs all of the medical clinics and hospitals throughout the country), the Canadian government has nothing to do with actually *delivering* health care services to Canadians. In fact, the vast majority of medical facilities, from hospitals to walk-in clinics, are privately run; they can choose their own staff, and decide how they want to deliver care to their patients, just like an American hospital. The difference is that the government pays for those services, not the patient.

The financial arrangements between the federal, provincial, and territorial governments and all of these hospitals and clinics can get pretty complicated, but from the viewpoint of the patient, it's fairly straightforward. When we go to a hospital or medical clinic, we just show them our health insurance card upon arrival. When we're discharged from the hospital (or when our doctor's appointment is finished), we simply walk out and go home; no bills, no paperwork.

Now, despite this, about two-thirds of Canadians get extra coverage that either they or their employer pays for. That's because, although Canadian Medicare covers a lot, it does fall short in some important areas.

For example, prescription meds are not covered by Medicare (although, to be fair, the government does use price controls to keep the cost of pharmaceuticals *way* down). On top of that, Canadians pay for their own dental care and prescription eyeglasses. Add in other things, like ambulance services, physiotherapy, and home care, and you can see some pretty large gaps in our basic coverage. In fact, government insurance only covers about 70 percent of a typical Canadian family's annual medical costs.

That's why many Canadians (or their employers) 'top up' their Medicare with a private insurance plan. Of course, as with private plans in the States, we run into the same barriers as our American cousins: pre-existing conditions may prevent us from getting certain coverage, and if we lose our job, we immediately lose any insurance benefits our employer provided.

Fortunately, even if we lose this extra coverage, Canadians still have that basic 70-percent coverage, so if a serious illness or injury occurs, we are guaranteed to have access to the health services we need. That's pretty much what happened to our family back in 2002. (Yes, we did have some supplementary insurance, but everything important was already covered, and when Kristen left the hospital after a six-month stay, we had absolutely no debt.) The bottom line for us was that, when it mattered, the government stepped in and looked after us when we were in the middle of a terrible medical crisis, so that we could focus on helping our daughter get better.

I've given you a really basic description here of how our health care system works, but if you'd like more information, I can recommend two good places to start:

- The Canadian Government's website [https://www.canada.ca/en/health-canada/topics/health-care-systems.html] offers a wealth of information on Medicare, prescription drugs, the different services we can access, and a variety of other resources.
- Wikipedia has a great page that describes both the history and present state of the Canadian Healthcare system [https://en.wikipedia.org/wiki/Healthcare_in_Canada], so that you can understand it in an historical context.

If these resources aren't enough, a Google search for "Canadian Health Care" will bring you a mountain of results. Still, I recommend that you start with the above two links, so that you have a solid base of knowledge before launching a more in-depth search.

Happy hunting!

And with that out of the way, we can begin our story…

PART I

Early Warnings

The Call

Many parents seem to view their kids with a mix of concern and fascination. We never stop caring or wanting to get involved in their lives (usually to their great annoyance). And of course, these days, it's hard to escape the dual role of "my kid's biggest fan" and "worrier-in-chief"—especially when you can pick up the phone or go online and get an instant update on every major event (and crisis) in your children's lives.

Here's an example. One night a few years ago, I was at home watching TV when my phone rang. I saw that it was my daughter Kristen, who was attending university at the time. The first thing I noticed was that she was calling me on FaceTime. This was odd, because normally, she would just text me or send me an email.

I took the call, and her first words were, "Dad, I don't feel too well."

When someone calls you just to tell you they're not feeling well, that's unusual. When that person also has a serious medical problem, it drifts into ominous territory. In Kristen's case, the problem was her kidney. It had been about ten years since she had received a new one in a transplant operation.

"I see," I said, trying to sound calm. "Where are you feeling bad, hon?"

"I feel kind of sick to my stomach. My kidney feels really hard, too."

That concerned me.

What made it even worse was that she was calling me from her university dorm room in Antigonish, a two-hour drive from our home in Halifax, Nova Scotia.

I took a silent breath. "Okay, do you have any other symptoms?"

"I think I might also have a fever."

Sore stomach, hard kidney, and maybe a fever. Alone, they didn't mean much, but together, they might be a sign her new kidney was having trouble.

In the ten years since her transplant operation, Kristen had been vigilant about her health, and she knew all the signs to watch for. But this knowledge could also work against her, and her mind could start to make up imaginary ailments on its own.

That's where a second opinion, even from a worried dad, could be very helpful. We carefully went through her symptoms again.

After a few minutes, I noticed that she had started to settle down, and so had the symptoms. When I asked her if she wanted to go to the nearby hospital, she said, "No, I'll wait till tomorrow and see how I feel."

We said our good-byes. I told her I loved her, and disconnected.

Now, alone with my thoughts, I felt my calm act begin to fall apart. The weight of the call, and the emotional baggage it carried, started to sink in.

It took me back to that awful spring ten years earlier when, out of nowhere, Kristen was diagnosed with end-stage kidney disease, and my wife Debbie and I nearly lost her. Once again, I felt overwhelmed by anxiety as I remembered the painful operations, dialysis treatments, drugs with their horrible side effects, and everything else we thought Kristen had put behind her.

Nervously, I sat and waited to hear from her again, but there was no second call that evening. Or the next.

And the next time we spoke, she told me that the problem wasn't to do with her kidneys at all (although it was still serious).

KRISTEN REMEMBERS…

I actually had a bladder infection that was turning into a urinary tract infection. I had to make an appointment with the campus clinic to be checked, and then have my prescription transferred from a pharmacy in Halifax to one in Antigonish.

Making that appointment meant seeing a new doctor, which is always stressful to me. To make sure I am properly treated, I have to go through my entire medical history first—and that's quite a lot of history.

Of course, while we'd been stumbling in the dark ten years earlier, now we knew what we were dealing with. Now we could properly diagnose a phantom pain and decide whether it required a hospital visit or a time of wait-and-see.

It was a bittersweet knowledge, though, because it couldn't undo all the needless trauma and pain that my daughter had had to endure.

* * *

Over the years, when I've shared our story with others, I've been shocked at how many people knew a friend or family member who also had kidney disease. And when I looked into the numbers, they confirmed what I was hearing: as of 2019, the U.S. Department of Health and Human Services estimates that more than *one in seven Americans*—about 37 million people—have chronic kidney disease (or CKD) in some form, from mild to end stage.

Knowing this, I was dismayed at how few people take it seriously, especially considering how it can impact your life and the lives of those who are close to you. CKD is a 'silent killer': as it slowly destroys your kidneys, they compensate by working harder, but they compensate so well that you don't even notice that they're failing. Physical symptoms don't start to appear until it's pretty late in the game, when your kidneys have lost about 50 percent of their capacity. And once that capacity's gone, it's gone forever. What makes this frustrating for me is that it's so easy to find out ahead of time whether you're at risk of CKD by getting a simple blood test, and yet most people don't seem to know about it.

With these thoughts in mind, I sat down to write the story you're about to read. I decided to focus on how the disease had affected us personally: the devastating effect it had on our daughter and our family, and the invaluable, hard-won lessons we took away from that awful time. However, over time, I noticed our story had become more than just a cautionary tale. The finished story also talks about the wonderful people who walked beside us on our difficult journey: the healthcare specialists whose caring and expertise made it possible for Kristen to return to a relatively normal, productive life, and our family and friends who offered their help and support in so many ways throughout the ordeal.

I had two main goals in writing this story: first, that it would give you, the reader, a better understanding of how dangerous CKD is; and second, that it would motivate you to do everything possible to avoid this terrible disease.

I hope that I succeed.

Remarkably Ordinary

(Early 2002)

Up until the spring of 2002, our lives had seemed remarkably ordinary. Debbie and I had both grown up in Halifax. We'd met through work—Debbie was a branch secretary at an insurance company and I worked at a family-owned insurance agency. We were married at St. John Vianney Church in Lower Sackville, at that time, a small community outside Halifax.

Kristen, the oldest, was born in 1987, followed by Danielle two years later, and Allison two years after that. We sent them all to Sacred Heart School in Halifax, vacationed as a family in the summers, and went through the usual challenges and joys, good and difficult times, that most families go through.

In 2000, when Kristen was 13, she was diagnosed with a minor heart disorder. Otherwise, she was just like her sisters, doing all right in school, and involved in different sports and social activities. Just a typical kid.

Because it wasn't serious, Kristen's heart disorder only required an annual checkup, along with a few lifestyle changes. For one, she had to take antibiotics before having her teeth cleaned at the dentist, so that bacteria from her mouth couldn't get into her system and cause a heart infection. She also had to quit the soccer team because we were told that too much running and jumping around could strain her heart.

Otherwise, it didn't really interfere with the quality of her life. In fact, in the two years that followed her heart diagnosis, she seemed relatively healthy and happy.

By early 2002, though, Debbie and I began to see a noticeable change in Kristen's behaviour. She was was becoming very moody and often seemed tired and withdrawn. She was also starting to miss a lot of school days, and her grades, which had always been good, were starting to slip. Her teachers were noticing, too. We were told that even when Kristen made it to class, she seemed to have a lot of trouble focusing on her work.

Because of all this, a grim possibility suddenly loomed on the horizon: Kristen might fail Grade 9. As any parent knows, falling a year behind doesn't just affect a child's educational track; it can also be devastating to their social life and self-esteem.

As bad as all this was, it was made even worse because we couldn't understand why our daughter was acting this way. It was like two different people were living in the same body. When I would drive Kristen to school in the morning, I'd almost have to drag her out of the house; when I would pick her up in the afternoon, she'd come running to the car as if everything were just fine.

Debbie and I were completely bewildered: how could Kristen feel sick and irritable when she woke up, and then be her normal, cheerful self a few hours later? Was she just being a moody teenager, was she acting this way because something was bothering her at school, or was it something else? Soon, our frustration boiled over into daily battles with our daughter.

KRISTEN REMEMBERS…

A typical day started with me throwing up and telling Mom and Dad I wanted to stay home. I missed a solid 20 days of school and my work was less than satisfactory, but I didn't care.

As we would find out later, people with advanced chronic kidney disease often display symptoms that seem to come and go for no reason. In Kristen's case, whenever we booked an appointment with her pediatrician, none of her symptoms would actually appear while we were there. The dizziness and nausea, the loss of appetite, the painful cramping in her hands that made her fingers stiffen until they were almost like claws—all would disappear by the time she saw the doctor. This meant that the best we could do was describe the symptoms from memory.

Unfortunately, the doctor wouldn't prescribe any tests for Kristen based only on our complaints. (Of course, not knowing what was wrong with Kristen, Debbie and I wouldn't have known what tests to ask for anyway.) So, despite our increasingly vocal demands for help, we were met with a brick wall of skepticism. When Kristen said that her vision was blurry, we were told to take her to an optometrist. When Kristen complained of having absolutely no energy in the mornings, we were told to make sure she got to bed earlier.

KRISTEN REMEMBERS...

I can remember one morning, sitting up in my bed at 7:00 a.m. with a dizzy feeling and a large knot in the pit of my stomach. I could barely move because I was feeling too nauseous even to stand.

My mom became angry with me, screaming for me to get up and get ready for school, but her words seemed like babbling noises, so I just ignored them. I grasped my bedside table and struggled to make my way to the bathroom. With every piece of clothing, I found it more difficult to get dressed. I found it almost impossible to button my shirt because having to look down made me feel even dizzier.

Finally I made it downstairs, taking one step at a time. My mom urged me to eat my breakfast but I snapped at her, saying that I wasn't hungry, that I would just throw it up in the end. I began to cry with frustration because I didn't know why I was feeling so awful.

We followed the doctor's orders, but nothing seemed to help. Of course, we were still dealing with symptoms, not the underlying cause. Had we known that kidney disease was the culprit, we would have dealt with it a lot differently. In fact, had we found out early enough, we could have started treatment for Kristen a lot sooner, and spared her a lot of the emotional and physical trauma that she went through over the following year.

But we weren't medical experts, and we didn't know what to look up online, or what books to read, or even what questions to ask in the first place. And as a result, we nearly lost our daughter.

Whenever I think back, it's painful to remember how hard we were on Kristen at the time. Not only was she having to cope with this terrible illness, but she was also getting no support from her family, her teachers, or her friends. The only feedback she got from anyone during that time usually took the form of criticism and anger.

KRISTEN REMEMBERS...

It seemed hopeless.

I felt sick, and my mom thought I was antisocial, my dad thought I was lazy and slacking, my doctor thought I was just being a teenager, and my teachers thought I was a bad student.

In March of that year, the situation would reach a new low when our family took a trip to what is, for many people, the happiest place on earth: the Walt Disney World Resort.

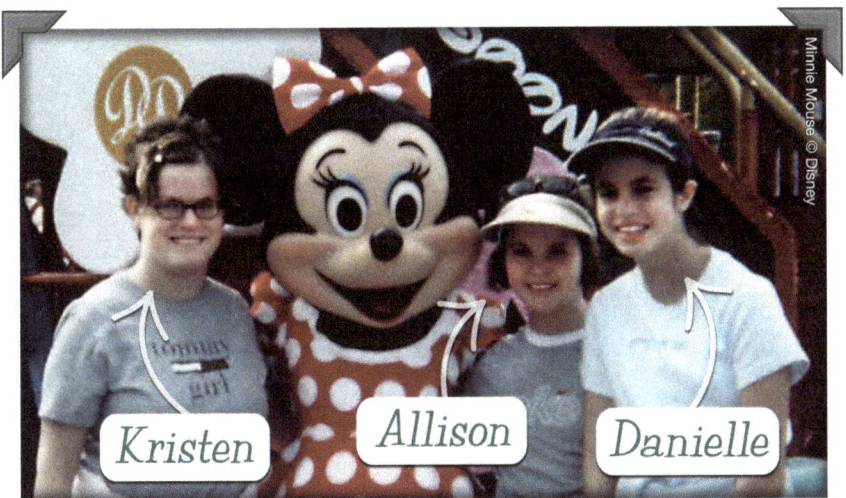

Group photo — with a new friend!

Spring Break

(March 2002)

Three months before March Break, on Christmas morning—after a lot of planning and saving—I had surprised the girls with reservations for an entire week at the Walt Disney World Resort in Florida. Since then, three very excited kids (and two equally excited parents) had been impatiently counting down the days until school let out.

Finally, the last day of classes arrived, and with a spring chill in the air, we packed our bags for a week in the Florida sunshine. We were booked on an early-morning flight, so we decided to stay overnight at a hotel near the airport. This ended up being a good decision, because the kids were all so nervous about the flight that none of them slept well, and we ended up rushing to catch the airport shuttle the next morning. Of course, their nervousness wasn't too surprising; this was their first time flying, so everything that Debbie and I saw as a routine part of travelling—from getting our luggage checked in, to going through security, to waiting for our boarding call—was new and exciting to them.

KRISTEN REMEMBERS...

I'm already a very anxious person; when it comes to travelling by plane, I STRONGLY detest it, even to this day. That morning, I woke up feeling nauseous and in pain, so the last thing I felt like doing was climbing out of bed, even if it was to go to Walt Disney World.

Soon after arriving at the airport, we were boarding our flight. Within minutes, we had all stowed our carry-ons and nestled into our seats. As the engines fired up, we all gripped the armrests for dear life, held our breath, and sank helplessly into our seats as the jet swept us skyward!

KRISTEN REMEMBERS...

As we were boarding the flight, the fact that I felt sick but didn't know why was compounded with my nervousness at being on a plane, to create a perfect storm of awfulness. I distinctly remember eating dry Corn Pops to have something in my stomach. I was so nervous that the nausea got the best of me, and when the pilot turned off the seat belt light, I immediately went to the bathroom and threw up.

That was how I started our family vacation.

A few hours later, we touched down at the Orlando International Airport in Florida. After renting a car, we drove to our destination, a wonderful resort called Vistana Villages. It was a beautiful complex, with a big pool in its centre.

In the days that followed, we happily traded our coats and boots for shorts and T-shirts, as we visited the sites and attractions, and relaxed by the pool in the evenings. There was even a bar and grill by the pool where you could enjoy a gourmet hot dog or burger, a fruit smoothie or iced coffee, and then dive back in.

KRISTEN REMEMBERS…

Every day, we overindulged in what Dad said were smoothies (but were actually virgin daiquiris), swam in the hotel pool, visited the attractions, and generally had a great time. Well, in the afternoons, anyway.

For me, every morning was sheer torture. I would wake up with my head spinning, sick to my stomach, and with a throbbing headache, and then start my day by running to the bathroom for an intense session of dry heaving.

Walt Disney World was, to put it mildly, amazing! All the different attractions were fantastic, and we had a wonderful time. For the most part.

As anyone who's been there knows, the trick is to arrive at the gates as early as possible in the morning, so you can take advantage of everything that the park has to offer.

That wasn't happening with us, though. Throughout our stay, we were never able to leave the villa before noon. This was because a certain slowpoke named Kristen had a lot of difficulty launching herself out of bed each morning.

KRISTEN REMEMBERS…

Mom and Dad were becoming increasingly frustrated with me because they thought I was being lethargic. Mom also thought I was being antisocial;

this added insult to injury because not only did I feel sick, but I also felt bad for making everyone wait.

It was just like at home: we would all wake up early, only to have Kristen get out of bed long after everyone else, and complain that she had a sick stomach. We'd try to get her to move, have a little breakfast, and around 11 o'clock, she'd finally start to come around and feel a little better.

By noon, we would finally be heading for the Walt Disney World Resort. By early afternoon, Kristen's mysterious symptoms would have completely disappeared and she'd be back to her old self again, leaving the rest of us baffled—and very annoyed.

KRISTEN REMEMBERS…

When we went to stay in a hotel at Clearwater Beach, I remember that it was so beautiful, and we should have had a really great time.

Instead, what I remember most is how my mom got sooooo mad at me because I didn't want to do anything. Finally, she became so frustrated that she told me I should have just stayed home. I know she felt really bad after the fact because to this day, she looks at pictures of me during the trip, and cries every time.

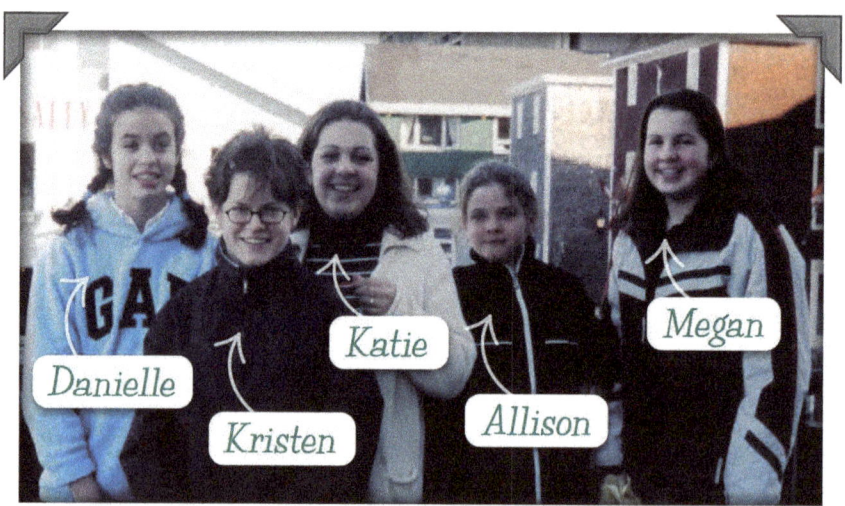

Visiting the Halifax Waterfront!

Heart Tests

(Wednesday, April 17, 2002)

A few weeks after our Florida trip, some friends in Michigan flew their girls up to Halifax to spend Easter weekend with us. We had known Megan and Katie's folks for years, and we thought that because they were close in age to our own girls, they would all have a wonderful time.

Unfortunately, that ended up not being the case. Just like our Florida trip, every day, before going anywhere, we would all have to wait for Kristen, who would sleep in and then take forever to get ready. And even when she was up, she seemed to have little interest in spending time with the other girls.

Now, when I look at group pictures from their visit, it's clear that something was wrong with Kristen. She'd lost a noticeable amount of weight, and although smiling, she looked tired. The progression of her disease had been so gradual that we hadn't noticed her fading away before our eyes.

One thing we did notice was that Kristen seemed to be constantly drinking water. At the time, we thought this was great, and joked that she would have the best skin of everybody in the family. What we didn't realize was that she was drinking so much because she was severely dehydrated; we would later find out this was another sign of kidney disease.

* * *

A week after Megan and Katie returned to Michigan, Kristen was scheduled to go for her annual heart checkup. Because she was still under 16, I took her to a cardiologist at the Izaak Walton Killam Health Centre. The 'IWK' was (and is) the largest children's hospital in the Maritimes, and we were very fortunate to live nearby.

Since Kristen's first heart diagnosis two years earlier, they'd been keeping tabs on a condition called *aortic insufficiency*. Although it wasn't life-threatening, it meant that her heart wasn't operating at full capacity.

When blood is pumped through your heart, it gathers oxygen and important nutrients that it will carry through the rest of your body. The last stop before it leaves your heart is a chamber called the *left ventricle*. From there, the blood is pumped out through a special opening called an *aortic valve*. Like the other valves in your heart, the aortic valve is supposed to open to allow blood to leave, and then immediately slam shut so the blood can't 'double back.' The sound of a normal heartbeat—'lub-DUB, lub-DUB'—is the sound these valves make when they close.

KRISTEN REMEMBERS…

In my case, the aortic valve only has two cusps instead of three, and so it is split down the middle. As a result, the blood does not flow properly from my heart. It has a 2-alternating-with-3 beat, and it sounds like a washing machine.

The left ventricle in Kristen's heart never completely empties of blood, and so it gets very crowded when the remaining blood combines with newly arriving blood. This causes two problems: first, the ventricle has to expand to make room for the extra blood, and second, her heart has to work harder to pump the blood out. This puts her at risk for both an enlarged heart and high blood pressure. It also causes her to get tired easily because her heart has trouble pumping that oxygen-rich blood out to her body where it needs to go.

KRISTEN REMEMBERS…

Because I have an irregular heartbeat, it restricts me from being able to do strenuous exercises.

One incident that I remember, quite vividly, was the week before my heart appointment, when Katie and I went for a run. I had to stop suddenly because I felt an extreme amount of pressure on my heart.

Kristen probably had this problem since birth, and it had gone unnoticed until her pediatrician had found it when Kristen was 13. Now, at 15, Kristen was meeting with the cardiologist for her third annual appointment.

KRISTEN REMEMBERS…
I now see them every two to three years, and they check to ensure the flow and leakage are still the same.

The cardiologist ran an echocardiogram and an ultrasound test. After the tests were done, Kristen joined me out in the waiting room. The doctor came out soon afterwards to give us some bad news: the tests showed that Kristen's heart was enlarged.

This was serious. An enlarged heart could mean that her blood pressure was too high. It could also be a sign of fluid buildup around her heart. Either way, if left untreated, it would eventually lead to heart failure.

Just to be sure, the doctor told us they would schedule a re-test. If the second test returned the same results, and showed that her heart really was enlarged, it could explain some of Kristen's symptoms over the previous six months, like her constant fatigue and oversleeping, and also the chest pains she'd experienced when she'd gone running with Katie.

But it wouldn't explain *all* of her symptoms: What about the nausea, the stiff and crooked fingers every morning, the weight loss? And why did the symptoms come and go?

We still didn't feel any closer to finding answers to these questions. But we now had more to offer the pediatrician than our own suspicions and stories. Now we had physical proof that something was very wrong with Kristen.

Pediatrician Appointment

(Thursday, April 18, 2002)

The next day, Kristen was scheduled for an appointment with her pediatrician. Looking back, I think her life was probably saved by the fact that her appointments with the cardiologist and pediatrician happened to be so close together.

That morning brought with it perfect spring weather: sunny and warm, with buds beginning to open on the trees. It should have been a pleasant reminder of the approaching summer; instead, it brought only worry, and on two fronts. First, although the previous day's tests had finally given us concrete proof that something was wrong with Kristen, we still had no idea what that something might be.

Second, we were very concerned about how much school she had missed. With her sick days piling up, another morning away from school would put Kristen even farther behind her classmates.

KRISTEN REMEMBERS...

When I was in school, I may as well not have been there at all because I couldn't focus on anything. I was usually exhausted even when I spent the day sleeping.

The first thing we discussed with the pediatrician was the cardiology test, and what the results could mean. Then the doctor asked Kristen a series of questions: "When did you start throwing up? When did the headaches start? Where are your headaches? Are you active? What's your diet like?"

Kristen described all of her symptoms, while Debbie talked about Kristen's unusual behaviour over the previous months.

KRISTEN REMEMBERS...

I was pointing to the various parts of my head where I often felt pounding sensations. We described my dizzy spells and my excruciating chest pains, and also how my periods had started to become irregular, and then finally stopped.

As I listened to all the routine questions, all I kept thinking was, "I'm missing school for this! I thought you were supposed to make me feel better."

The doctor then asked Debbie and me to wait outside, and talked to Kristen some more.

KRISTEN REMEMBERS…
When my parents left the room, the doctor asked me: "Are you pregnant?"
I was puzzled by the question, and could only respond, "Um, NO!!" I hadn't even thought about boys yet, and going to an all girls' school really limited the opportunities for any potential pregnancy.
I was told, "Well, you're just a teenager and maybe you have a bit of social anxiety."
I felt dazed and confused, and had no idea why I was there. I only knew that I was 15, but I felt like I was withering away inside.

Before we left, the doctor gave us a requisition for blood work. Something about what we discussed (probably the heart test) must have struck a chord.

KRISTEN REMEMBERS…
It was only after hearing about my test results that the doctor jumped on lab work, because it isn't normal for a 15-year-old girl to have an enlarged heart.

We left the office thinking, "Finally!" We were now moving forward, and would soon start to get some answers.

At the same time, I knew that getting her blood work done the next day would mean three mornings in a row of missed classes. Kristen seemed fine, so I decided to take her to school, and postpone the blood work until Monday.

It was a decision I would regret later.

Blood Work

(Monday, April 22, 2002)

First thing Monday morning, I drove Kristen to the IWK hospital. We arrived at 6 a.m. so we wouldn't have to wait too long when the blood clinic opened at 7. Even that early, a lot of folks were already in the waiting room when we got there. Fortunately, when the clinic finally opened and we registered at the front desk, we only had to wait a few minutes before a phlebotomist came in and called for Kristen.

KRISTEN REMEMBERS...
Up to that time, any appointments with my pediatrician were usually around 10 a.m. or later, and by that time, my symptoms were pretty much gone. The morning I went in for blood work, we got to the hospital when I was still feeling my worst, all achy and nauseous. The phlebotomist noticed immediately.

After Kristen left with the phlebotomist, I sat alone in the waiting room, thinking about how we had arrived at that moment.

By this time, it had been about six months since we'd started noticing a change in Kristen's behaviour. Now, along with her being more irritable and depressed, her symptoms—painful cramping in her hands and feet, terrible headaches, and bouts of nausea and fatigue—were lasting longer and becoming more severe.

Worse, if the last appointment with her doctor had been anything to go by, there was no guarantee we would even find a connection between all of these symptoms.

Looking back, there's a horrible irony to the situation. The whole reason we chose a pediatrician over a family doctor was to ensure that all our kids would get the best possible medical care. From a practical viewpoint, it made sense: if you have a problem with your car's brakes, you take it to a brake specialist. In the same way, you'd expect that the best person to take your kids to would be a doctor who specializes in children's health.

Years earlier, we had started with an excellent pediatrician, who was there when Allison, our youngest daughter, was born, and who looked after her and her older siblings for several years. However, when that doctor retired, a new one took over the caseload.

At first, everything was fine. In fact, it was the new doctor who discovered Kristen's heart condition. This was why Debbie and I sided with the doctor for as long as we did when Kristen started to show her first symptoms in late 2001. But, as these symptoms grew worse, and our complaints continued to fall on deaf ears, we became more frustrated with the doctor's inability to help our daughter.

Now, after months of getting nowhere, I sat in a hospital waiting room, still feeling bewildered and anxious, but at least a little hopeful. I had no idea what these tests would find, but I knew that we were finally taking some sort of action.

KRISTEN REMEMBERS...

They did a full lab test, full blood work. They checked for EVERYTHING.

A short while later, Kristen came out, a small bandage taped to her arm. Once again, she said she didn't feel well, and so I drove her home instead of to school, angry that she was falling yet another day behind her classmates.

KRISTEN REMEMBERS...

The phlebotomist had made a comment that I looked very sick and it was only for that reason that Dad took me home. It was nearing the afternoon, and so I was bouncing back to normal. Dad yelled at me, saying that the smile on my face made him mad and if it wasn't for the blood lab lady, I would be going to school.

Blood Test Results

(Tuesday, April 23, 2002)

The next morning, we sent the girls off to school, going through the motions of a normal day, even though it was starting to feel anything *but* normal.

KRISTEN REMEMBERS...

That morning I was feeling dizzy and exhausted as I tried to cope with another day of school. I had an excruciating headache and could only wait for the afternoon to come because that's when the pounding usually stopped.

But this time it didn't stop. This time, it continued to get worse. Everyone was asking if I was okay because I looked as white as a ghost. I just wanted to go home.

The pediatrician called later in the morning. Apparently, the test results had come back showing some kind of problem related to Kristen's kidneys. Something called her creatinine level was much higher than it should be.

So, what did that mean? Before I could ask, I was told we had to take Kristen to the IWK hospital the next day for more tests.

"What kinds of tests?" I asked.

The pediatrician didn't offer any specifics, but said that Kristen could be there for as long as a week. I was told to take her to the sixth floor of the IWK—they would be expecting us.

The sixth floor? I wondered. What was up there?

The doctor recommended that we wait until mid-morning to avoid the early-morning shift change by the nursing staff. (As I would later find out, shift changes are often the most chaotic time at a hospital.)

As I hung up the phone, I felt reassured. We would finally be getting some help for Kristen, and from specialists working at a top-notch hospital.

Needless to say, I was surprised when we got another call a short while later, this time from the IWK: No, we were absolutely not to wait until mid-morning; we were to bring Kristen in first thing.

Bewildered, I hung up the phone and told Debbie about the call. As I held her, she started to cry. I also began to tear up, feeling my own anxiety start to build. Was this an emergency, or not? What had the test results shown?

KRISTEN REMEMBERS...

As I waited for Dad to pick me up from school, I felt so faint and dizzy. When I got into the car, Dad was unusually silent. He seemed very worried about something, but he didn't say what. Did someone die? I wondered.

We entered our driveway, and when I got into the house, Mom and Dad sat me down at the table. They told me that my doctor called, saying I had to go into the hospital the next morning.

I tried to keep myself from crying, and I tried to remain strong, but the thought of why I was going into the hospital kept whirling through my mind. What about school? I couldn't fail Grade 9! And what about the dogs? Abby and Alex couldn't live without me!

I was scared.

I called my friends and told them I wasn't going to be in school the next day. They asked why and I said, nonchalantly, because I had to go into the hospital. I said I didn't think I was going to be in there for long, that it was probably only going to be a few days. Little did I know.

Meeting Dr. Crocker

(Wednesday, April 24, 2002)

Early Wednesday morning, I drove Kristen and her mother to the IWK hospital. When we got there, we were directed to the "6 North" Clinic. We took the elevator to the sixth floor, and stepped out into the hallway.

A sign near the elevator showed that 6 North treated kidney disease, cancer, and blood disorders in children. I felt a cold sensation creep through my stomach. What were we doing here?!

When we got to the nurses' station, Debbie and I were given a lot of paperwork to fill out: insurance information, medical history, allergies, medications Kristen was on, and so forth. When that was done, the nurse put an ID band on Kristen's arm, and we were introduced to the health care team who would be looking after her.

KRISTEN REMEMBERS…

Much to our shock, we were greeted by basically the entire sixth-floor doctor and nursing staff.

A nurse escorted us to a small room opposite the nurses' station, and told us that we would be meeting with a kidney specialist.

I was confused. A kidney specialist? I remembered the pediatrician mentioning a possible problem with Kristen's kidneys. But your kidneys were just responsible for filtering out stuff that your body didn't need. What could her kidneys have to do with the range of problems that Kristen had gone through over the past six months?

A few minutes later, a man entered the room and introduced himself as Dr. John Crocker. I'll never forget my first impression of this wonderful fellow. With his thick eyebrows and receding, bushy hairline, he immediately struck me as a kinder, gentler version of Oscar the Grouch from *Sesame Street*. Otherwise, he was in pretty good shape for a guy in his mid-60s.

After sitting down with us, Dr. Crocker didn't waste any time: "Kristen is in renal failure and it is life-threatening."

The cold sensation in my stomach from earlier now grew into a frigid chunk of ice. I shook my head, trying to grasp what he was saying. Life-threatening? How could a problem with her kidneys be life-threatening?

I felt sick. Not even a week earlier, we had sat in the pediatrician's office and been told that Kristen was probably fine, just a "typical teenager." Now, another doctor—a specialist—was telling us that Kristen's life was in serious danger.

As Dr. Crocker described what was happening to Kristen, a lot of things suddenly began to make sense: her mysterious, come-and-go symptoms, her mood swings, her extreme weight loss. In stunned silence, we listened as he told us what Kristen's blood work had revealed. One thing I vividly remember was learning why her creatinine level was such a big deal. As Dr. Crocker explained, Kristen's creatinine should have measured under 100, but it was actually over 1500—15 times the normal level. He said this meant her kidneys were functioning at only 10 percent their regular capacity.

KRISTEN REMEMBERS…

The normal range for two healthy kidneys is 50 to 100; mine was actually 1700.

While Debbie and I sat in shock, Kristen appeared calm, taking everything in. At one point, she looked over at Debbie and said, "Mom, everything will be all right." Looking back, I still don't know whether Kristen's calm demeanour was a result of her not understanding the seriousness of her situation, or just being relieved to know what was causing her to feel sick. Maybe both.

KRISTEN REMEMBERS…

My biggest concern was missing school. I remember asking Dr. Crocker, "What am I supposed to do about school, because I have a test in a couple of weeks."

He responded, "You don't need to worry about school, you just need to worry about getting better."

Dr. Crocker told us that, because her kidney damage was so severe, Kristen would be starting treatments immediately, and so she would be going in for some surgical procedures the next day. He also said that she would be in the hospital for a lot longer than a week.

KRISTEN REMEMBERS…

The sixth floor of the IWK would end up being my home for the next six months.

As we discussed Kristen's symptoms and her treatment options, Dr. Crocker assured us that he would be open with us every step of the way, and that we would be told everything we needed to know to make the best decisions for our daughter. It was such a relief to hear him say this. Although we knew Kristen's condition was serious, we also felt like she was in competent hands.

Looking back, I think of that first meeting as our "ticket to ride"—climbing onto an emotional roller coaster that, over the coming months, would drop us into a dark valley one day and lift us skyward the next. Through it all, though, it was good to know that Dr. Crocker and the IWK staff were there with us.

PART II

Fight for Survival

Surviving

During that first meeting with Dr. Crocker, we were shocked to learn how close Kristen had come to dying. In the coming days, we would also learn that although she was now in a hospital, surrounded by qualified specialists and dedicated staff, she wasn't out of danger yet. In fact, her battle was really just beginning.

The previous months had left Kristen physically and emotionally drained, and now she would have to find new reserves of strength just to survive. Her frail condition also meant that every option that her doctors considered for treatment would be overshadowed by complications.

One of the biggest challenges now was to undo some of the damage caused by her failing kidneys. Specifically, they would have to bring two things under control: her electrolyte balance and the concentration of urea in her bloodstream.

When your electrolytes are balanced, this means they're within a certain range of concentration—not too high, not too low. Electrolytes like sodium and potassium help your cells to function properly, keep your muscles working, move fluids to where they're needed around your body, and do a lot of other life-sustaining work. When your kidneys stop working, your electrolytes fall completely out of balance. This means that none of these important jobs get done, and you end up getting very sick.

When your kidneys are healthy, they also divert a lot of waste products out of your system—with urea being one of the most toxic. Normally, urea gets filtered out by your kidneys and then leaves your body as urine. When your kidneys shut down, though, the urea level starts to rise in your bloodstream, and when it becomes really concentrated, you develop a very serious condition called *uremia*.

KRISTEN REMEMBERS...
The urea level is supposed to be between 1 and 8; mine was at 48.

Uremia and an electrolyte imbalance had been the worst culprits behind many of Kristen's symptoms over the previous months. Slowly and silently, they had stolen her strength and destroyed her ability to think clearly, until she was unable to function in school and was often left bedridden. They had made her so sick and nauseous that eventually she couldn't keep any of her food down, so that by the time she was admitted to 6 North, she had lost a dangerous amount of weight.

That wasn't the worst of it, though: if her urea concentration kept rising, we were told that Kristen could eventually slip into a coma; and even if they managed to revive her, she would probably end up with permanent brain damage. To stop that from happening, Kristen would now have to be fast-tracked for a series of procedures so that they could begin treatment right away.

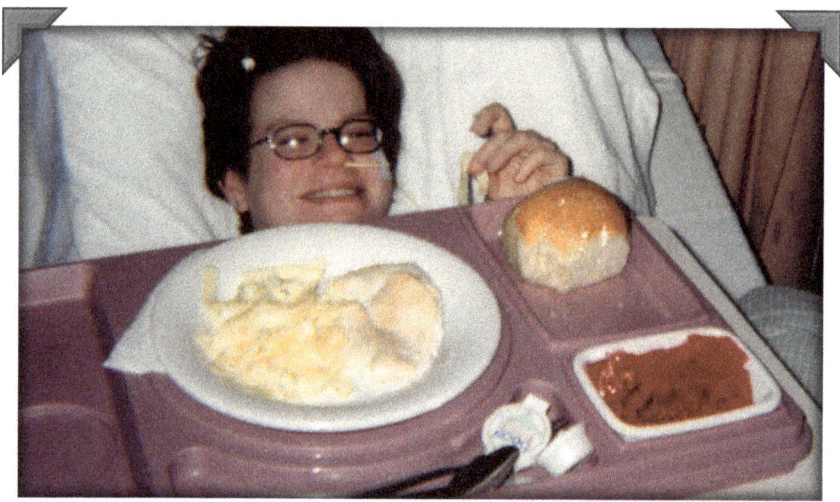

Hospital food sucks!

Settling In

(Wednesday, April 24, 2002)

Like many diseases, chronic kidney disease is progressive. In its early stages, where your kidneys start to lose some of their function, you don't show any symptoms at all; the only way you know you have it is through a test that measures your creatinine level. By stage 3, where your kidneys are functioning at about 50 percent, you start to experience minor symptoms, and your doctor will usually recommend changes in your diet and lifestyle to slow the disease down. When you reach stage 5, or *end stage*, where your kidneys have basically stopped working, it's time to think about dialysis treatment or getting a replacement kidney.

When Kristen was admitted, she was well into stage 5.

Now that we understood what that meant, and that she would probably be in the hospital for several months, Debbie and I would spend the next few days scrambling to get up to speed.

There was a family room on the sixth floor that had some computers, so we immediately began to contact friends and family. In the coming months, many of these people would become our pillars of support, helping us not just on a practical level, but emotionally as well.

KRISTEN REMEMBERS...

Basically, my mom and dad got a hold of our entire support system to ensure we had plenty of people around us. Mom got in touch with some of my aunts to ask them to help out with the house, look after my sisters, and so on. Dad contacted my uncle and aunt in New Hampshire, and they came up and stayed for a week.

After Kristen was settled in, Debbie and I returned home to pack what she would need for the next few days. Later that afternoon, I picked up Danielle and Allison from school. I told them their sister wasn't well, and that she would be staying at the IWK hospital for a while.

KRISTEN REMEMBERS...
I don't think Danielle and Allison understood everything that was happening, but they knew that I was in the hospital, and they were worried that they were going to lose their big sister.

When we returned to the hospital, we learned that Kristen would have to be put on a special diet. Because so many kinds of food would knock her electrolyte levels out of balance, for her survival, she had to cut out practically everything she was used to eating. Any foods with potassium were especially off-limits.

KRISTEN REMEMBERS...
Because my body was in complete shutdown, I was not permitted to eat anything with high potassium because my heart would have gone into cardiac arrest. So, my first hospital meal was a tuna sandwich on white, with cranberry juice and Jell-O.

We were also surprised to learn that Kristen's pediatrician had stopped in to see her.

KRISTEN REMEMBERS...
I only saw my pediatrician once during my stay, and it was on the day I was admitted. I was sitting up in my bed getting poked with a needle for an IV. The doctor came into my room, saw me sitting there bright red with anger and fright, and said, "How's the food?"
I felt disgusted, thinking that instead of a little sensitivity, or an apology, or at least a little bit of concern, all I was asked was, "How's the food?"
After that, my pediatrician left.

That night, Kristen slept in a hospital room, attached to monitors and an intravenous drip, and surrounded by strangers instead of her family. It also felt strange for us, not having our daughter at home, and although there would be many nights like this in the weeks and months ahead, we would never get used to it.

The Biopsy

(Thursday morning, April 25, 2002)

Early the next morning, Debbie and I dropped Danielle and Allison at school and returned to the hospital. When we arrived at Kristen's room, she and Dr. Crocker were already going over the day's schedule.

As we found out, it would be a hectic one, starting with her first medical procedure. Although the doctors were pretty confident that Kristen's kidneys were too far gone to save, they had to be sure; this meant she needed a kidney biopsy.

They started by taking an X-ray to find the exact location of her kidneys. Then, after applying a local anesthetic on her back, directly above one of the kidneys, they used a special needle to pull out a small, spaghetti-shaped tissue sample.

KRISTEN REMEMBERS...

The best way I can describe the experience is with a great Canadian reference: a slap shot in hockey. That sound the puck makes when it hits the goalie's glove? Imagine what that feels like for the glove, and you'll get a sense of the severe pressure and unpleasant pounding sensation that your kidney experiences when the needle goes in.

Your kidneys move whenever you breathe. This meant that each time they took a sample from Kristen's kidney, she would have to keep still and hold her breath until the needle came back out (which would take about 30 seconds). If she were to move or breathe during that time, it would ruin the sample and they'd have to take another one.

Dr. Crocker wanted to make sure he was taking good samples, so the first one was immediately sent to the pathology lab and quality-tested.

When the lab called back to confirm the sample, they asked, "Why did you send us a kidney sample from a cadaver?"

There were dozens of terrifying moments and close calls in the months that followed, but this particular one runs a chill down my back whenever I remember it.

* * *

With the first sample approved, Dr. Crocker took the remaining samples he needed.

Now, specially trained lab technicians would carefully study the samples under a microscope and try to determine the exact condition of Kristen's kidneys (though the call from the lab had already solved that mystery for us) as well as what may have caused them to fail.

Labs typically process samples on a first-come, first-served basis, so patients usually don't see their biopsy results for about a week. Of course, because Kristen's case was so serious, Dr. Crocker fast-tracked the lab work so we would get the results the next day.

They had finished the procedure at around noon, and by one, Kristen was back in her room, recovering. She now had to stay in bed for the rest of the afternoon, while the nurses kept an eye on her. They needed to watch for post-op complications, which could range from a fever, to a lot of pain around the biopsy site, to blood in her urine.

Or, in Kristen's case, to the urine being completely blocked. Soon after the biopsy, her kidneys started producing blood clots the size of golf balls, and before long, she couldn't pass urine at all.

KRISTEN REMEMBERS...

It was the most unsettling and excruciating pain and discomfort ever. Imagine when you need to pee, you feel like you're ready to burst, but there's a plug in the way. It was AWFUL.

To help her pass urine, they inserted a catheter into her bladder. This released the pressure almost immediately, and—needless to say—she was soon feeling a lot better.

Of course, her day was still only half-finished: another procedure was scheduled for that evening, and this one would be a little more complicated.

Dialysis Catheter

(Thursday Evening, April 25, 2002)

Like the biopsy, Kristen's second procedure of the day should have been done weeks—or even months—earlier, when her kidneys were still functioning. Now, with no time left and her system crashing, they had to put in a dialysis catheter immediately so they could start treatment. In other words, we were in the middle of a worst-case scenario.

If we'd known sooner, the doctors would have had more options available, in terms of both the kind of dialysis treatment they could use and how they could prepare Kristen for it. In terms of treatments, a few months earlier they would have had a choice between hemodialysis and peritoneal dialysis.

With *hemodialysis*, your blood is cycled outside your body into a machine called a *dialyzer*. The dialyzer acts like a kind of artificial kidney, filtering out wastes and excess water before returning the blood back to your system.

With *peritoneal dialysis*, or P.D., your tummy is filled with a special solution called *dialysate*. While the dialysate rests there, it draws waste products and excess water from your bloodstream and into your tummy. After a few hours, the dialysate is drained out, taking all the waste products and extra water with it.

The treatment they ultimately chose for Kristen was peritoneal dialysis. This was because of her serious condition and the short amount of time they had to prepare her for treatment. Hemodialysis would have required that one of Kristen's veins be artificially strengthened so that it would be able to accommodate massive amounts of blood flowing out to, and in from, a dialyzer. The way they strengthen a vein is by attaching it to a nearby artery. This causes a lot more blood to flow through the vein, and after several weeks of increased flow, the vein becomes strong enough to handle hemodialysis treatment. But Kristen needed treatment immediately, which meant we didn't have several weeks to wait while one of her veins built up enough strength. That left us with P.D. as our only option.

Of course, P.D. offers its own challenges: like hemodialysis, it also requires an entry-and-exit point, and so it also involves surgery and a healing period (although P.D. surgery is generally simpler and the healing time shorter). To prep you for peritoneal dialysis, they need to insert a length of tubing called a *catheter* into your lower stomach. They run the catheter right into your peritoneal cavity, and then stabilize it so it doesn't move around. Treatment usually begins after the stitches around the catheter have had time to heal, usually about two weeks. During treatment, the catheter is hooked up to a special machine called a *cycler*. The cycler moves fresh P.D. solution into your tummy, and later, it draws that solution out again, along with waste products and extra water.

Although peritoneal dialysis has a simpler start-up procedure than hemodialysis, it does have a higher risk of infection: we were told that if the catheter site leaked, Kristen might end up with peritonitis.

On top of all these complications, we had another problem: the procedure for putting in a catheter usually requires that you be put under. This isn't a problem if you're still a healthy weight, but Kristen had lost about 30 pounds over the previous six months, and she was now considered anorexic.

KRISTEN REMEMBERS...

The healthy weight for a 15 year old at my height is between 90 and 120 pounds. When I was first admitted, I weighed in at just over 75 pounds.

Because of her condition, there was no way she could endure a general anesthetic—only a local would be possible. And, as we found out, the only type of P.D. procedure that could be done using a local was *percutaneous* (or "through the skin").

KRISTEN REMEMBERS...

As I was wheeled down to the operating room, I was so scared. I didn't know what to expect and my mom was terrified for me. We were told that I wasn't able to go to sleep for the surgery because I would go into immediate convulsions from being so malnourished.

For a percutaneous operation, they start by making a small incision near your belly button. Then they use a special guide wire to run a catheter tube in through the incision, and they feed the catheter in and down, until the tip is settled at the base of your tummy.

After that, they make a tiny incision from inside your tummy at the spot where they want the catheter to come out. This is called the *exit site*. (In Kristen's case, the exit site was a few inches to the right of her belly button.)

When the incision is made, they run the other end of the tubing out through the exit site. Then they close up both the first incision and the exit site, and they run saline solution through the catheter to test it for leaks.

Finally, the part of the catheter tubing that comes out through the exit site is sealed at the tip with a special adaptor, and a clean dressing is put over the exit site.

KRISTEN REMEMBERS...

They gave me a dose of medicine to make me "happy," but that didn't take away the pulling, tugging, and painful sensations that I felt as they put the dialysis catheter in.

After the surgery, I felt a sense of relief because, as I said to my mom, I didn't want to go through that again. I was in excruciating pain.

The procedure was finished by about 7:30, and afterwards, Kristen was wheeled back to her room. She was in a lot of discomfort ("kind of like being punched in the stomach a thousand times," she said) and soon fell into a much-needed sleep.

Under normal circumstances, the exit site would have at least two weeks to scar and heal before dialysis began. In Kristen's case, her 'healing time' would have to be measured in hours instead of weeks, because the treatment had to start as soon as possible.

* * *

Afterwards, I dropped Debbie and the girls at home. When I returned to the hospital later that evening, Kristen was still sleeping.

No surprise there. Not only had she gone through two gruelling procedures in the same day, but she'd also had nothing to eat since the previous night—and that was only a half-slice of bread, with a bit of salt-free spread and some jam.

I sat in a nearby waiting room, and watched a hockey game to pass the time. Around midnight, I checked in to see if she was awake, but she was still sleeping soundly.

I was actually glad for this: after all Kristen had been through, she was finally surrounded by caring and knowledgeable people, and was able to heal and recuperate in peace.

Feeling pretty tired myself, I headed home to catch a few hours of sleep.

Biopsy Results, Dialysis Begins

(Friday, April 26, 2002)

When Debbie and I returned to the hospital the next morning, Kristen was still asleep, so I went to the family room to send out a few emails and update everyone on how things were going. A little after nine, Debbie came to tell me that Kristen was finally awake.

When we met with the doctors, they told us that Kristen would have to start taking a special protein drink to help bring her weight up.

KRISTEN REMEMBERS...

I couldn't eat, so they had to give me a protein drink called Nepro, which had 1900 calories in every shake. I had to drink three a day; it tasted metallic, and with every gulp I cringed as it slowly went down my throat.

Later, when the lab results came in from her biopsy, they just confirmed what we all knew: Kristen would need a transplant.

* * *

Although Kristen would mostly be recuperating that day, she was also scheduled to start with some limited dialysis 'exchanges.' The plan was to run small amounts of dialysis solution at a time, and if these were successful, to increase the amounts.

Because the catheter site had barely begun to heal, there was a high risk of a fluid leak, an infection, or both. We could only pray there would be no serious complications.

We were also hopeful, though. If it worked, the dialysis would do the same job her kidneys would normally have done. Of course, where her kidneys had once cleaned her system and balanced her electrolytes using hundreds of thousands of tiny, specialized filters, the dialysis treatment would rely on dialysis solution and her peritoneum to do the same thing.

Before starting the dialysis session, a nurse checked Kristen's temperature. This was necessary because it would warn them if she was running a fever. This, combined with cloudy urine, could be a sign of infection. If that happened, they would have to stop her dialysis and put her on antibiotics until the infection was gone. Given how badly she needed dialysis at that point, this would be a disaster.

Fortunately, her temperature was normal, so they turned on the cycler, prepped the bags of dialysis solution and the lines to and from the cycler, and hooked up Kristen's catheter to one of the lines.

Since this was her first exchange, there was no old dialysis solution to drain out, so they just released fresh solution into her tummy. This step is called the *fill time*, and normally it takes about 10 minutes; because Kristen was starting out with just a small amount of solution, it only took a minute or so.

This was followed by the *dwell time*, where the dialysis solution sat in her tummy and drew toxins and excess water out of her bloodstream. Dialysis solution is mostly made up of sterile water, but it also includes other important stuff that will help you feel better. This includes electrolytes like sodium and potassium, and a type of sugar called *dextrose*. The dextrose is what pulls all the water and waste products out of your system; the more concentrated the dextrose, the more it draws out.

Usually, the dwell time takes about four to six hours. In Kristen's case, a small amount of solution was used, so the dwell time—like the fill time before it—was much shorter than normal.

After the dwell time, they drained out the old dialysis solution. Then, as soon as it was completely drained, they ran fresh solution into her tummy, and a new exchange began.

Over the next few days, this process was repeated over and over again. Because of this, Kristen spent the entire weekend hooked up to the machine.

KRISTEN REMEMBERS...

I was on the dialysis machine 24 hours a day. My legs turned to mush because I wasn't mobile; I was constantly lying in bed because I wasn't permitted to move while they were doing exchanges.

This is why astronauts have to use bikes in space to maintain muscle mass. Mine wouldn't be used much over the next month, so they soon lost their tone and strength.

Although Kristen was pretty exhausted from the treatments, she did have some brighter moments. Two of her schoolmates stopped by to see her, which really lifted her spirits. We were also pleasantly surprised when a couple we knew, Randy and Maureen, dropped off a lovely casserole—a wonderful and thoughtful gesture.

We were all pretty frazzled by the events of the previous week, but Debbie and I felt very lucky to have our daughter at the IWK hospital, being looked after by such great doctors and staff. While everybody complains about paying taxes, we were seeing first-hand the wonderful health care system those taxes pay for.

Meeting Dr. Acott

(Saturday, April 27, 2002)

At that time, there were actually two doctors on 6 North who specialized in pediatric nephrology. We'd already met Dr. Crocker when Kristen was admitted. On Saturday, the second specialist on the team, Dr. Philip Acott, stopped in to see how she was doing.

She was still very sore from the catheter operation, but that was to be expected, he said. What did concern him was her loss of appetite.

Along with the Nepro, they were trying to feed Kristen sandwiches, Jell-O, turkey and rice, and a few other items from a very limited menu of 'safe' foods. It all looked pretty good to me, but because her uremia was making her nauseous, she just wasn't able to keep any of it down. This meant they'd have to consider an unpleasant option: if Kristen couldn't eat or drink anything the normal way, she would need to have a feeding tube inserted through her nose so the food could go directly to her stomach.

Another serious problem she was dealing with was a condition called *uremic acidosis*. Acidosis is pretty common among kidney patients. This is because one of the jobs your kidneys are responsible for is filtering out things like phosphate and sulphate, which make your blood more acidic. When your kidneys stop working, and the concentration of acid rises, one way your body compensates is by leaching calcium out of your bones to reduce the acidity. Over time, this can cause a condition called *osteopenia*, or reduced bone mass. If this isn't treated, it can lead to *osteoporosis*, where your bones become brittle and easily broken.

So, there were now two reasons why dialysis was so important to Kristen: by treating her uremia, it would bring back her appetite, and by balancing her electrolytes, it would stop her bones from becoming brittle.

To help restore the calcium she had already lost, the doctors decided to start her on a calcium supplement. Like Nepro, it was definitely an acquired taste. Although they try to make these drinks taste good—in this case, like a chocolate milkshake—when you compare an artificially flavoured medical supplement to a real, honest-to-goodness milkshake made with chocolate syrup and ice cream, there's really no contest.

That evening, my parents took Allison and Danielle out for dinner so that Debbie could stay with Kristen, and I could go home and take care of the dogs.

The poor little things were lost without Kristen. While I typed up some emails to friends and family, Abby sat beside me, looking absolutely forlorn. The previous night, Alex had slept in our room, but kept getting up and going to Kristen's room, where both he and Abby usually slept. It was heartbreaking, but there was no way to explain to them what was happening.

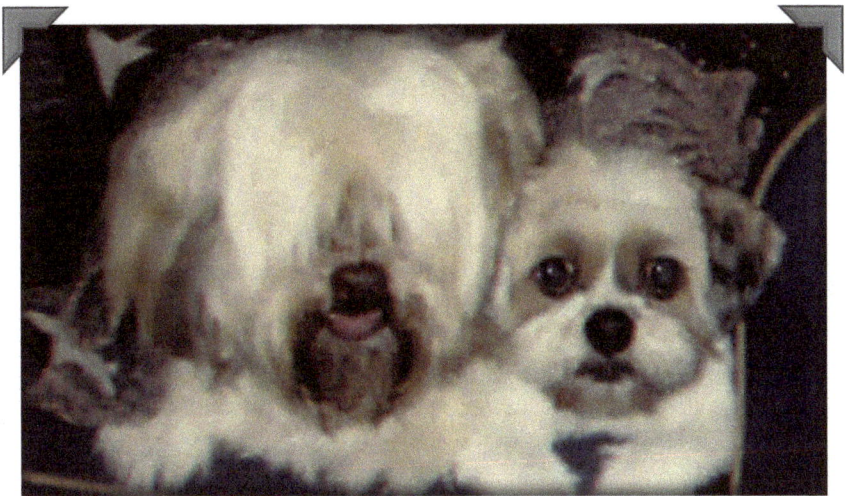

Kristen's buddies — Alex and Abby!

Day of Rest

(Sunday, April 28, 2002)

Sunday thankfully turned out to be a day of rest for our family. Kristen still felt some pain from the operation, but thanks to the dialysis, she was finally able to eat a little bit.

Emily, one of her friends who'd been in on Friday, stopped in again that afternoon. We were really touched that she would take the time to come and visit Kristen, especially knowing how much it eased Kristen's loneliness to see a friendly, familiar face.

Debbie's friend Theresa, who had been her maid of honour at our wedding, took her to a performance of 'Stars on Ice' in the afternoon—a much-needed break. Debbie's mom, Bertha, also stopped in with a homemade apple pie for the ward nurses. To my dismay, they swooped in like vultures, leaving none for me!

That evening, my parents came to visit Kristen, and to take Danielle and Allison out for dinner again. This was the first time Dad had seen Kristen since she'd been admitted, and he got all choked up, couldn't say anything, and had to walk out of the room. (I was relieved that he hadn't seen her on Thursday or Friday, when she'd looked much worse.) In a reversal of roles, I put my arms around him and did my best to calm him down.

Mom, on the other hand, took it in stride. She gave Kristen a hug, and told her everything would be fine and that the people at the IWK would take great care of her.

That evening, Kristen asked me to stay with her, so after I dropped off Debbie and the girls at home, I came back and spent a few more hours at the hospital. At 11, I headed home again, as I had to be up early the next morning, in time to get the other girls off to school.

Debbie and I were also scheduled for another meeting that morning—with a transplant nurse. Because Kristen was in end-stage kidney disease, we would have to begin looking for donors immediately.

Meeting the Transplant Nurse

(Monday morning, April 29, 2002)

Now that we were searching for a kidney donor, the IWK brought in a special transplant nurse to help us. As we were to learn, finding a replacement kidney can be a daunting and emotionally draining experience; without their help, I don't know how we would have done it.

Our appointment with the nurse was almost as overwhelming as our first meeting with Dr. Crocker. She covered a lot of ground, describing the transplant procedure and donor requirements, and getting us up to speed on the challenges that lay ahead. It was stuff you would normally have months to think about; we were getting a crash course in a few hours.

She told us that because of Kristen's condition, they would have to fast-track the process of finding a living donor from among our family and friends. This meant we would have only two weeks to find someone before they were forced to begin searching for a deceased donor.

We had hoped it would be possible to find a living donor for Kristen. I had assumed that a family member would be the best bet, and from what the nurse told us about donor requirements, I was right. However, the more I learned about the selection process, the more I realized how challenging it would be, even from within our own family.

Basically, you have to meet three requirements before you can be a donor. I was relieved to find out that I met the first one.

KRISTEN REMEMBERS...

In order for me to have a transplant, I needed a donor, so my father stepped up. He had the same blood type as me and was willing to do anything he could to save my life.

The first thing they look for to match—blood type—was in our favour: Kristen and I were both type O. (For kidney compatibility, + or – doesn't matter; type O is type O.)

Interestingly, because I was type O, it meant that I could donate a kidney to practically anyone, whether they were type O, A, B, or AB. This made me a 'universal donor.'

But there was a flip side to this: because Kristen was type O, she could only receive a kidney from somebody else who was type O. Granted, it's the most common blood type, with about 47 percent of the population being either type O– or O+. But this also meant that 53 percent of the population would be disqualified before we even started looking.

The second test was for something called HLA typing. An HLA is just a special protein that helps your body's immune system to locate and attack invaders.

With HLA typing, there are six markers that doctors look at to see if two people match. Three of these markers come from your mother, and three from your father. This is why your family members are usually the best prospect for a transplant: their markers are more likely to match yours, and so their donated kidney is less likely to be attacked by your immune system.

The third test, cross-matching, is a blood test that checks to see if your body will reject the donor's tissue. This is the big one: even if a donor passes the other two tests, a bad cross-match means it's game over—no transplant from them, and your search begins again.

We also learned that it made quite a difference whether the donor was living or deceased.

KRISTEN REMEMBERS…

Everyone kept telling me that it would be better to get a kidney from a living donor because the chances of keeping it were better.

The nurse told us that 'living' was the better option, for a few reasons. The first was compatibility: a living donation was most likely to come from a family member, and as I mentioned, family members would be more likely to match Kristen. The second reason was red tape: with a deceased donor, Kristen could end up waiting years for a compatible kidney to become available. Even then, the deceased person's family would have to give their consent to the donation; a series of tests would be needed to make sure the kidney was both healthy and a good match; and, of course, there might be people ahead of Kristen who were also a match for that kidney.

The third reason was timing. We were told that one of the biggest challenges in getting a deceased kidney actually comes from scheduling the operation. For obvious reasons, this can't be planned in advance, so you have to be ready at a moment's notice in case one becomes available. This means your life could be put on hold for years. With a living donor, you can set up a time when both you and the donor are ready for the operation.

The fourth reason was longevity. On average, a living donor kidney will last much longer than a deceased donor kidney. (This is important because recipients generally live longer than their donated kidney.) A deceased kidney will last an average of about 14 years, while a living kidney will average about 26 years, nearly twice as long. Interestingly, this also means that if they have two possible living donors to choose from, they will choose the oldest donor first; this is because the younger one is statistically more likely to be healthy enough to donate a kidney 15 or 20 years down the road.

After the meeting, the nurse gave us some pamphlets and other material to read, and we sat together, absorbing all this new information and pondering our chances of finding a match for our daughter.

Meanwhile, Kristen was facing another serious problem that needed immediate attention: despite the dialysis, she still didn't feel much like drinking her protein supplements. As Dr. Acott had warned us, an unpleasant procedure loomed on the horizon.

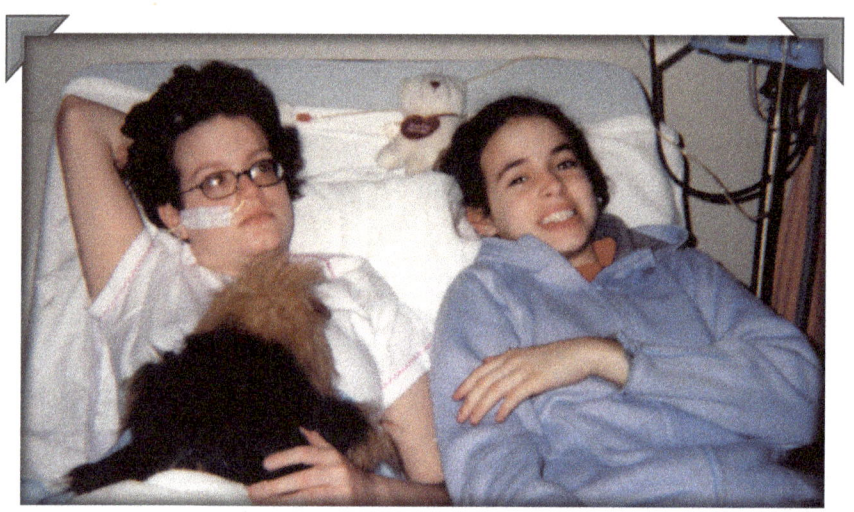

Not the best of days.

Nose Tube

(Monday afternoon, April 29, 2002)

After a weekend of nonstop dialysis exchanges, Kristen was finally given a few hours away from the machine on Monday afternoon. This was also her first chance to get up and walk around since the catheter had been put in on Thursday evening.

We were told that if her dialysis continued to progress and she was feeling well enough, then in a few weeks she might be able to escape the sixth floor for an hour or so, and head outside. Our plan was to arrange a visit with Abby and Alex in the courtyard, as this was the only place on the hospital grounds where dogs were allowed.

It might seem odd that, with Kristen only being in the hospital a few days, we would already be talking about things like courtyard visits and spending time with pets. However, we knew that making these kinds of plans would give Kristen something to look forward to, a future goal to help her get through those days when she was being poked and prodded and stuck with needles, or just those moments when she was feeling down or lonely.

This was a particularly bad day, because although the news was good on the dialysis front, she was still having a lot of trouble drinking the Nepro. If her weight didn't go up, a transplant operation would be impossible. It would be major surgery, requiring that Kristen be put under for several hours, and there was no way she would survive such a long operation at her present weight.

The only solution was to use a feeding tube.

Needless to say, Kristen wasn't impressed.

KRISTEN REMEMBERS...

It was one of the most uncomfortable sensations I experienced in the hospital.

The name for this procedure is *nasogastric intubation*, which sounds about as unpleasant as the actual experience. If you've ever had one, you'll probably remember it—vividly if there were complications.

Basically, it involved running a plastic tube up through her nose, down her throat, and into her stomach. To help reduce friction and chafing, the nurse applied a dollop of gel to the end that went in first, and also gave Kristen a cup of water, which she drank in small gulps to help the tube slide down more easily. When it was in, the nurse put an adhesive bandage on Kristen's nose to secure the tubing so it wouldn't move around or get pulled back out.

After the procedure was over, they still had to keep an eye on Kristen in case there were any complications. These could range from skin irritation to nausea and even stomach cramps; not exactly a Christmas list for Santa, but she would now finally be able to take in some nourishment.

Or at least, that was the plan. Unfortunately, fate had other ideas, and would hit us with a series of minor disasters that would once again cause her health to crash and her numbers to climb.

Searching for a Donor

(Tuesday, April 30, 2002)

Tuesday actually started on a positive note. First, the doctors ran some tests to see if Kristen still needed the bladder catheter that they had put in after the biopsy. They injected fluid through the catheter and found that the flow rate was normal, and whatever had been causing the blockage was gone.

End result: Kristen—one. Bladder catheter—zero!

We were also told there was a slim chance that, if everything went okay for the rest of the week, Kristen might be able to return home for an hour or so over the weekend. We were all very excited by that possibility, however remote it might be.

In the morning, I visited my doctor to get the forms for my blood work. Afterwards, I left the forms at the nurses' station so they could confirm that no tests had been left out.

In our meeting with the transplant nurse the previous day, we'd already crossed a lot of potential donors off our list. Although I was still on the list, I was starting to realize that the first hurdle, compatible blood type, wasn't so much a way to help find a matching donor, as it was to clear the field. If you had the wrong blood type, you were kicked off right away. If you had the right blood type, it only meant you stayed on the field a while longer, until the next round of tests.

In the following days, the call would go out to family and friends that Kristen was in need of a kidney transplant, and that we would be grateful to anyone with the right blood type who was willing to be tested as a possible donor.

We would find our relatives and friends to be very supportive, and many of them would volunteer to be tested. Still, although I kept it to myself, I was beginning to feel a heavy weight bearing down on me. Seeing your child dying before your eyes, and being helpless to do anything, is one of the most frightening and painful experiences you can imagine. Also one of the loneliest, because it's something you really can't share.

I prayed that we would be able to find a donor from within our own family, and that if it wasn't one of us, it would at least be someone we knew.

As I was finding out, though, regardless of all your plans and your best efforts, most of what happens in life is completely beyond your control.

Dialysis Stopped

(Friday, May 3, 2002)

The next two days passed quietly by, marked by a series of small changes for the better. Kristen's dialysis exchanges were gradually increased, and her numbers started to come down. Also, despite her lack of appetite, she was now getting nutrients into her system through the feeding tube.

We slowly began to fall into a comfortable rhythm, feeling a sense of progress with each dialysis exchange.

Until Friday.

Shortly after midnight on Friday morning, Kristen's catheter started leaking dialysis fluid during an exchange. By 5 a.m., they realized that the leaking wasn't going to stop on its own, and so her dialysis was put on hold.

To make matters worse, later that morning, her feeding tube began to clog up. When this happens, the nurses try everything possible to unblock the tubing. Otherwise, they have to replace it with a new one, an experience that is both time-consuming (for the nurses) and unpleasant (for the patient). The nurses did all they could, from flushing the line with Coca-Cola to forcing air into the tube. Unfortunately, nothing worked—whatever was blocking the tubing wouldn't budge. So, with her throat still raw and irritated from the first procedure, Kristen had to have the old tube pulled out, and a new one put in.

As expected, the experience was far from pleasant, and when it was over, Kristen also had to endure a common side effect: an excruciating headache.

The nurses told us that problems with feeding tubes and dialysis catheters are not uncommon. Still, this was cold comfort to poor Kristen, who had to deal with both problems on the same day!

* * *

On the family front, things were much better: Kristen received a funny get-well card from Katie in Michigan—it made us all laugh, and was a much-needed release after the stress of the previous week. That afternoon, our friends John and Maureen (nicknamed "Sully and Moe") arrived from New Hampshire, after a nine-hour drive. They would be an incredible source of support to us over the following weeks and months.

A surprise package also arrived from a good friend of mine who lived in Baltimore, Maryland. His name is Alan, but we've always called him "Buster," and he's like a third grandfather to the kids. After hearing about Kristen, he'd called me a few days earlier to find out what might pick up her spirits. "Well," I'd said, "anything to do with Disney would be wonderful."

I thought he might send up a doll, or a piece of Disney memorabilia. Instead, here was this great big box that must have weighed about twenty-five pounds.

When Kristen opened the box, we were all stunned. It contained a huge collection of Disney-related stuff: videotapes (remember those?), a beautiful water globe, dolls, books, and colouring supplies!

* * *

One of the first things Sully and Moe did after arriving was to make Kristen's calcium treatments more pleasant. Along with the calcium shakes she had to drink, she was also taking Tums—two a day—to help increase her calcium intake. Not surprisingly, the selection at the hospital was limited to the no-nonsense regular flavour.

KRISTEN REMEMBERS...

Tums are loaded with calcium, but to make sure I got all that calcium into my system, I wasn't allowed to take them with food. So, I had to take my Tums and then wait about an hour before eating (which didn't make much difference to me because I had no appetite).

My Uncle John and Auntie Maureen brought up these fancy Tums from the United States that were cleared with the doctors, and they tasted like pink peppermints ☺

Sully would also be instrumental in helping me to lose some weight. I was very worried that either my blood pressure or my weight would get me kicked off the donor list, and when I told him how difficult it had been for me to control my eating, he decided to take on the role of "diet police" to help me. I was determined to do whatever was necessary to move to the top of the list, and so I happily accepted his help.

The next day, I would have a breakfast of Special K cereal, a bagel with some diet peanut butter, and a half glass of orange juice; a lunch of beef veggie soup and another bagel; and a dinner of leftover Heart Smart lasagna with a low-fat homemade muffin. By day's end, I would come to realize that this was going to be a very, very tough haul.

* * *

Around noon, the resident surgeon came in to check the stitches around Kristen's catheter. He decided to keep her off dialysis for the weekend, to give the stitches more time to heal around the opening. If that worked, there would be no need for another operation to add more stitches.

The downside of putting her dialysis on hold until Monday was that it would once again send her numbers up and throw her electrolytes off balance, with all the problems that entailed. Everyone was disappointed by this setback, but the doctors had no other choice.

By late afternoon, we were relieved that Kristen's painful headache had finally gone and she was resting comfortably. However, by that evening, her creatinine level had crept back up to 1026.

On the Up-and-Up

(Saturday, May 4, 2002)

All patients on 6 North have their own room. This gives them some privacy when they have visitors or they just want to rest. When they're feeling up to it, though, they usually like to hang out with the other kids in the teen lounge or the family room.

Since the surgeon's visit on Friday, Kristen had been pretty much confined to her room, and was even discouraged from getting out of bed. This meant she wasn't just getting a lot of privacy, she was also getting pretty isolated.

On top of having to be by herself, she began Saturday morning with a low-grade fever. This was worrisome because it could be a sign of infection around her catheter. At the same time, her creatinine level had climbed to 1096—a lot lower than when she was admitted, but still almost 11 times what it should be.

The catheter itself still hadn't stopped leaking, but one of the nurses found something that gave us a little bit of hope: after taking a close look, she'd noticed that a weight at the end of the hookup was pulling down the catheter tube. Could this have been causing the leak? They released the hookup to loosen it, and we all crossed our fingers that this would solve the problem.

By Saturday evening, Kristen was feeling better, and her fever had gone away. Unfortunately, her creatinine level was now climbing past 1200. With no guarantee that her dialysis would be continued in the next few days, the 1700 reading we thought we'd left behind loomed ahead of us once again.

Blessed Boredom

(Sunday, May 5, 2002)

Like any calm before a storm, Sunday was wonderfully quiet and uneventful.

When the nurses changed the dressing around Kristen's catheter, it no longer appeared to be leaking. If it still looked good on Monday, we were told they would restart dialysis. They also removed her IV because she was now getting both food and fluids through the nose tube.

One surprising development was Kristen's creatinine level, which had actually gone *down* by three points from the previous day! Although we suspected it had something to do with her new feeding tube, nobody could really explain how it would stop her creatinine from climbing.

Meanwhile, I was looking forward to Monday, when I would finally be getting my blood pressure tested. This would be the first in a battery of tests whose results would hopefully keep me on the donors list.

I was now two days into my diet, and Sully seemed happy with my progress (although I wasn't too excited about the daily menu). One thing I was concerned about was that once Sully went back to New Hampshire, I would lose an important ally in my weight-loss battle. Still, despite my lingering doubts, he seemed pretty confident that he'd be able to keep an eye on me, even across that distance.

In the days that followed, I would see just how resourceful my old friend could be.

* * *

That afternoon, a few more visitors came by to see Kristen. One of her classmates dropped in, along with Bertha and Debbie's sister, Evie. Kristen's godfather, Rusty, also stopped by. He was a good friend of mine from back in university and now worked for the Tourism Industry Association of Nova Scotia. He was on his way to Antigonish to evaluate a hotel, but wanted to stop in before he left.

That evening, Debbie took Danielle and Allison to see a performance of the Lipizzaner Stallions. It was something the girls had really been looking forward to, but more importantly, it was an opportunity to just spend some time with their mom, away from everything else that was going on.

Another Day in 'Paradise'

(Monday, May 6, 2002)

By the end of Sunday, we still had high hopes that Kristen would be able to avoid a second catheter procedure.

On Monday morning, those hopes were dashed.

Around midnight, Kristen's catheter started leaking again—and much worse than on Friday. It looked like adjusting the weight on the catheter hookup hadn't fixed the problem after all. This meant the doctors would now have to operate.

They scheduled Kristen for surgery at 2:30 that afternoon. We were told that because the procedure would only take about 20 minutes, they would be able to use a general anesthetic. This meant Kristen would be able to sleep through it.

Kristen was very annoyed about having to go through the operation again, and blamed herself for the catheter not working. But, as the doctors pointed out, this happens in about three out of every ten cases. Kristen just happened to be one of the unfortunate 'three' instead of one of the lucky 'seven.'

Debbie and I were allowed to accompany Kristen and the surgery team to the OR floor so we could stay with her until they went in. Unfortunately, when we arrived, they found out there was a backlog of other patients already waiting for surgery. They didn't want to send us back to our floors, so we all waited until our turn came; it sort of felt like we were airplanes waiting on a runway for takeoff.

Soon, it was time for Kristen to go, and she was wheeled down the hall to the OR.

As she disappeared around the corner, I was suddenly struck by a terrifying thought: What if I never saw my daughter alive again? Frightening questions tumbled through my mind: With all the weight she'd lost, could she survive a general anesthetic, even for 20 minutes? What about other unexpected complications? Would there be a problem with the catheter? With the stitches?

Unable to protect Kristen, I felt that overwhelming sense of helplessness and dread begin to return. Afterwards, as Debbie and I sat in the waiting room, every possible complication played and replayed through my mind—after all, each development up to now had only led to some new complication.

Sitting there, I felt trapped. Who could I talk to? Debbie had enough on her plate, and I couldn't burden her with any more. And who else would understand?

I sat in silence, counting the passing minutes.

* * *

After an eternity, a nurse popped her head into the waiting room: the operation had gone fine, and we could now go in and see Kristen.

She was still sleeping when we got to the recovery room, and so we sat and waited with her. When Kristen woke up, she was not a happy camper. Although they had given her Tylenol and morphine, the post-op pain was pretty bad. Still, it was so good to see that she had made it through.

The doctors told us that they could only give her a day to heal before putting her back on dialysis; time wasn't on their side, and they would have to restart her treatment as soon as possible. That morning, her creatinine level had been close to 1300; now, more than 12 hours later, we knew it must be well above that.

Grace under Pressure

(Monday, May 6, 2002)

Early on Monday, before Kristen had gone into surgery, I was outfitted for my blood pressure test. It had been a week since we'd met the transplant nurse, and we now had only a week left to find a donor from among our family and friends. If none of us qualified, Kristen would have to be added to a national waiting list for deceased kidney donors.

Although many of our friends and family members had come forward, for practical reasons, we couldn't all be tested. Instead, they had looked at our medical histories, and narrowed the list down to the candidates most likely to be accepted.

Some had been struck off immediately because they weren't the right blood type. Others were ruled out because of health issues: my brother had problems with his liver, Debbie had already had kidney stones, and on it went. Out of everyone who had volunteered, there ended up being two strong matches: Debbie's nephew, Gary, and me.

Gary had just returned from a military posting, serving our country in Europe. Now he was stepping up to help family. He not only had the correct blood type, but he was also young and healthy.

Because I was older, they decided to run tests on me first. I was very relieved at this, and also confident that I would end up as the donor, because I was her dad and likely to be a good match.

That morning, they attached a blood pressure monitor to my arm. Over the next 24 hours, it would check my blood pressure every hour during the day, and every two hours at night.

This would tell them whether I had a problem with my blood pressure, or whether it just peaked at certain times (like when I thought about how much was riding on the results of, say, a blood pressure test!).

Looking back, I have to admit it was a very convenient way to be tested, but at the time, it just felt like another hurdle I had to climb so I could move on to the next bunch of tests.

Thrown from the Train

(Tuesday, May 7, 2002)

The next morning, I dropped the blood pressure kit off at the hospital. Afterwards, Debbie and I met with the surgeon, and he explained to us why Kristen's catheter had been giving her so much grief. Apparently, there's a membrane that covers your stomach muscles in front. If a dialysis catheter has to go in, this membrane can cause problems, so they usually remove a section of it beforehand.

Although not in Kristen's case.

Two weeks earlier, when they installed the catheter during the first operation, they'd been forced to use a local anesthetic because of Kristen's condition, and so they weren't able to remove the membrane.

This time around, they put Kristen completely under using a general anesthetic, and so they were able to take out part of the membrane without causing her a lot of pain.

Kristen still had some post-op discomfort, but it wasn't as bad as the first operation. Of course, she still didn't feel like eating, but when your tummy feels like it's just been used as a punching bag, you generally don't.

* * *

With Kristen's catheter now fixed and stable, and the lab people processing my results, there wasn't much for me to do, so I decided to take in a round of golf.

Over the coming months, the golf course would become a much-needed sanctuary for me, a few hours' break from the constant stress that seemed to come from every direction.

I actually felt pretty good that morning, and was excited about moving on to the next step as a donor. I was even getting used to my new diet: I had two apples on the course, with a lot of water, and I was looking forward to the chicken stir-fry that Debbie would be preparing that evening.

Halfway through the course, I stopped to call Debbie at the hospital to see if she'd heard anything. She mentioned that my brother Richard and his wife Judy had been in around noon to visit Kristen. Then, after a pause, she gave me some heartbreaking news: according to the test results, my blood pressure was too high. I had been thrown off the donor train.

I was devastated. Over the previous week, my anger and frustration at what my daughter was going through had been balanced by the thought that I could at least be a donor. Now, even that hope was gone. I couldn't provide for my daughter at a time when she desperately needed my help, and the culprit was the excess weight that I had carried all my life. My morale, which had already been pretty low, now hit rock bottom.

As a father, you never want to fail your kids, and I knew that I had failed Kristen. Still, not wanting to show anyone how I felt, I put on a brave face, and tried to pretend it didn't bother me.

Meanwhile, I could only watch helplessly as another lifeline was plucked from my daughter's grasp, and pray a new one would come from somewhere.

PART III

If at First You Don't Succeed...

Support System

Being thrown from the donor train was a frustrating and painful experience. Knowing that my failure was completely down to me made it even worse.

We had to carry on, though, and so I focused on helping Kristen in every way I could.

I had recently sold my interest in the family business to my brother, and I no longer worked there. This meant I was technically between jobs, so I now had a lot more time to look after Kristen than I would otherwise have had. To this day, I am convinced that the timing was divine intervention because it allowed Debbie and me to not only take care of Kristen during her hospital stay, but also look after things at home.

With Kristen out of immediate danger, we had also begun to play the long game. This meant that over the following weeks and months, Debbie and I would need to work alongside the hospital staff, closely involved in the day-to-day care of our daughter. Their expertise and hard work would restore Kristen's health so that she could survive a transplant operation; our love and attention would help her stay positive and focused on the future.

As we would find out, in some ways, this would be more difficult than dealing with the daily crises of the previous two weeks; a low level of anxiety and stress would be our constant companion, and Debbie, Kristen, and I would all have bad moments—sometimes stretching into hours, and even days—that would often push us to our emotional limits.

Throughout this time, the hospital staff were an enormous help to us. In the months that followed, I developed an incredible respect for the doctors, nurses, and support staff of 6 North. With a calm and professional demeanour, they took on everything, from daily snafus with IVs and nose tubes to life-or-death battles in the operating room. A patient's health might depend on the turn of a scalpel blade, or the correct type and amount of a drug, or spotting some subtle change in behaviour that could spell disaster if not dealt with in time—and whatever the situation, these people had to be ready for it, at a moment's notice.

Watching them go through these daily, often thankless trials with such compassion and skill, I could only see them as heroes.

* * *

Meanwhile, our lives moved on: While other kids were finishing their school year and looking forward to summer vacation, Kristen was now focusing on getting her weight up in the event that a kidney became available. In the following weeks, Debbie and I would try to make Kristen's stay more comfortable by surrounding her with things from home, and we would take on a lot more of the responsibility of caring for her.

At the same time, Gary was now stepping up as the next volunteer on our donor list. Would he be the one? We could only wait and see.

The Diet Police

(Wednesday, May 8, 2002)

By Wednesday, Kristen had been back on dialysis for about a day, and we were finally watching her numbers start to come down again.

With the drop in her numbers, Kristen's nausea began to dissipate, which in turn led to her appetite finally returning. Because the nose tube didn't interfere with her ability to swallow, they decided to give her some solid food. That afternoon, she enjoyed a peanut butter and banana sandwich, some French fries, a fruit cocktail, and a whole bunch of water. (Of course, I would know she was completely back to normal when she felt like eating first thing in the morning, but still…)

It was now my turn to not feel like eating. I was bitterly disappointed in myself for not only failing the test, but also throwing the responsibility onto my nephew Gary.

And it all came down to my weight.

All my life, I've struggled with it. Diets have always been tough for me because I find it difficult to give up what I like (everything, basically). Sully knew that, and was doing his best to help me with my new diet. Unfortunately, by the time I'd strapped on the blood pressure monitor that Monday, I'd only had a few days of low-calorie meals under my belt, not enough to make any real difference.

In the back of my mind, I knew that the odds of my being allowed back on the donor train were practically nil. But I also knew I had nothing to lose by trying, especially with Gary now being the only person standing between Kristen and the deceased donors waiting list.

One thing I didn't know was that a wonderful group of people were also determined to help me meet my goal. The first time I noticed their efforts was later that week. I was talking to some other parents on the floor, and one of the wives mentioned having some leftover scallops. Before I could get a word in, one of the nurses jumped in and said she was a deputy with the diet police and I was not to have any.

Without me knowing, Sully had been setting up a support network to make sure I didn't weaken. He'd already deputized some of the nurses, but that was just the beginning; over the coming weeks, the diet police would seem to appear out of nowhere. Friends and family would suddenly turn up, like angels on my shoulder, and make sure I didn't give in to the temptation of a second heaping helping, or a delicious dessert, or some other high-calorie treat.

They would even follow me to the golf course. One day, after having played nine holes, we went to the canteen at the turn. When I walked up to the wicket, the girl who served us immediately announced that the diet police had been in contact with her, and asked her to make sure that I stuck to my diet.

It turned out that Sully had found out my weekly golf schedule, and had called all the way from New Hampshire, to spread the word around the club. I just shook my head, rolled my eyes, and got an apple and a drink. After the round, we went up to the '19th hole,' only to be informed that they were also watching my choices. I couldn't overeat even if I wanted to!

So, instead of roast beef, mashed potatoes, French fries, ice cream, and all those other comfort foods I would have indulged in, I was now eating bagels, pita sandwiches, salads, and soups, and drinking water and milk.

I also started walking. On Wednesday morning, despite the fact that I absolutely hate exercise of any kind, I decided to walk the three-and-a-half kilometres (just over two miles) from our house to the IWK. Hearing this, Debbie gladly offered to bring the car to the hospital later that day, so that we could drive home together afterwards.

* * *

Later that day, Debbie and I had a chance to confirm something that had been weighing heavily on our minds: because Kristen had developed chronic kidney disease, was it possible that Danielle and Allison were also at risk?

You need a doctor to give you a requisition for blood work, but we had already decided not to go back to the girls' pediatrician. After asking around, we were surprised to learn that the mother of one of Danielle's classmates was a pediatrician! When we asked her if she could help us, she generously took the girls on as her patients.

A few days later, we took Danielle and Allison to their first appointment with their new doctor. By the end of the appointment, she had completed requisitions for them. As we left the office, I felt an incredible sense of relief knowing that we had found someone who we both knew and could trust. Immediately afterwards, requisitions in hand, we took the girls to get their blood work done.

Around 9 p.m., the pediatrician called to give us some good news: Danielle and Allison were healthy, with no signs of kidney trouble! After the emotional roller coaster of the previous few weeks, just having this off our plates helped us to sleep a lot easier that night.

A Hat Trick of Good Days

(Thursday, May 9, to Saturday, May 11, 2002)

That week, Gary began his donor tests, starting with blood work. With few other prospects, we could only pray that he would be a match.

Over the next few days, Kristen continued to feel better. She was chipper, cracking jokes, and eating everything they put in front of her.

Her catheter was working perfectly now, so the nurses were able to continue upping the amount of dialysis solution each day. By Thursday, her creatinine count had dropped below 1000 for the first time in almost a week, and her urea number was also out of the danger zone.

That evening, after taking Debbie and the kids home, I returned to spend a few more hours with Kristen. I was pleasantly surprised to find out that some other people had stopped by to spend time with her: Debbie's brother Jimmy and his wife (also named Debbie) had stopped in earlier, and so had my brother Richard and his wife Judy.

* * *

Kristen's teachers and classmates also pitched in to help cheer her up. We were amazed at how thoughtful they were.

KRISTEN REMEMBERS…

My class did a huge card and everyone signed it.

I also had teachers visit me and bring little trinkets. At the time I loved to do friendship bracelets, so my teacher Mrs. Driscoll brought me a giant bag of the string I needed.

I remember that some of my teachers were a bit remorseful when they came to visit. Some of them had been pretty spiteful towards me because I'd seemed to be so lax about my work. It was an eye-opening experience for them, that things aren't always as they seem.

* * *

On Friday, the doctors came in with the head surgeon and told us that if Kristen continued to improve, she might be ready for a transplant by July. They also told us that because she was doing so well, and Sunday was supposed to be a nice day, we might finally be able to take her down to the front courtyard of the hospital for a picnic.

Kristen couldn't wait because it meant that, after spending the past three weeks inside the hospital, confined mostly to a single room, she would not only be able to go outside, but also spend some time with Abby and Alex. Of course, there were caveats: she would have to be taken down in a wheelchair, and while she was there, she would have to be very careful not to make any sudden movements that might loosen the catheter. Still, the list of conditions could have been a mile long and she wouldn't have cared; she was going to see her dogs again!

We got another piece of good news: if Kristen continued to feel better over the next few days, then on Monday, they would let her try to drink the protein shake again. If she was able to drink it without feeling sick, then the "hose in the nose" might finally come out!

* * *

On Saturday, Kristen had no visitors, which was actually a good thing because she was able to get some quiet time. She was also on a four-hour respite from the dialysis machine, so to help get her muscles back in shape, we had her walk around the ward.

The positive developments of the previous few days had really lifted our spirits, and Debbie and I went home feeling pretty good. We were looking forward to Sunday and our first big outing as a family, even if it was only to the front of the building.

Although it was a good day, it also ended up being a busy one, so we didn't get to bed until after midnight. I fell asleep almost as soon as I hit the pillow—only to be awoken again a few hours later by the phone.

"What now?" I thought, as I frantically picked it up. The person on the other end of the line said he needed to speak to me, but I didn't recognize his voice.

Kristen had seemed fine when we left, but that had been hours ago, and any number of things could have happened since: Had her dialysis catheter sprung another leak? Was her nose tube blocked again? Had her nausea returned to kill her appetite?

Then he told me why he was calling: he was with the firm that handled security for the company where I had worked. Apparently, an alarm had gone off, and although it turned out to be nothing, they still had to phone someone with the company to let them know. My name hadn't been removed from the list of contacts, and, as luck would have it, I was at the top of that list.

My mouth felt dry as I thanked him. I hung up the phone, lay back down, and stared at the ceiling. Tired as I was, sleep didn't come for a while.

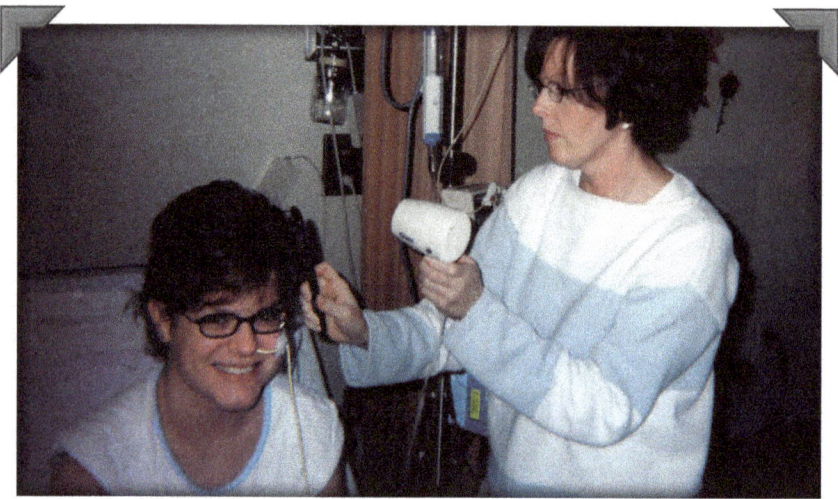

Getting ready to go outside!

Mother's Day

(Sunday, May 12, 2002)

Despite the progress we'd made over the previous few days, Sunday started off badly. This time, the crisis struck at home.

Debbie had a moment before leaving the house: blaming herself for not picking up earlier on Kristen's symptoms, and feeling overwhelmed by a million thoughts of how things could have gone. The fact it was Mother's Day probably didn't help.

We both seemed to have a lot of those moments—fortunately, not at the same time. A week earlier, I was sitting at the computer in the 6 North family room, writing emails to friends and updating them on Kristen's progress, when suddenly I began to well up over the enormity of what we were dealing with. Debbie had been nearby on the phone and saw what was happening. She immediately hung up the phone and came over to console me.

Now, it was my turn to console her. Debbie's thoughts that morning were triggered by something Kristen had said the previous night: how she wished she could go home and sleep in her own bed and have the dogs with her, and how all that had been taken from her.

Over the coming months, Debbie and I would often be overwhelmed by emotions that seemed to come out of nowhere, feelings of helplessness, frustration, and depression that were triggered by the smallest things. That morning, I knew I couldn't go down that route, so I concentrated on getting the dogs into the car, and Debbie and I drove off to see our daughter.

* * *

When we finally got to the hospital for the big visit, we found Kristen in high spirits and very anxious to visit with Abby and Alex. Part of the reason she was feeling so good was that her numbers were continuing to improve. Her creatinine had dropped below 850 and her urea level was also down.

Debbie helped Kristen wash and style her hair, and the nurses unhooked Kristen from the dialysis machine. Then we helped her into a wheelchair and headed downstairs.

After I wheeled Kristen into the courtyard, I left her and Debbie to fetch the dogs from the car. When I brought Abby and Alex to the courtyard, they needed a little time to get used to their strange new surroundings. When the courtyard finally met with their approval, they sniffed Kristen out, and had a wonderful reunion.

That day, the hospital was having a barbecue in the courtyard: hamburgers, hot dogs, salads, and dessert. Kristen didn't eat much, but with the diet police nowhere in sight, I suffered a moment of weakness. After my strict diet of the past week, this was like heaven. I did try to eat the healthier items, but I sort of lost points on volume. Afterwards, I promised myself I'd climb right back on the diet wagon the next day.

Although the weather had started out nice, fog soon began to roll in. Kristen was heartbroken about having to part company with the dogs, so we promised that we would try to arrange a visit the following week.

The visit made it clear how homesick Kristen was becoming, so we decided to see if we could make her hospital room more comfortable. Because every patient had their own room, families were encouraged to bring in furniture and other things from home so that it might feel warmer and less sterile.

KRISTEN REMEMBERS…

I ended up bringing a lot of stuff from home into my room. I had my blankets, and my nana bought me a feather bed because at the time the beds were extremely uncomfortable.

I had pictures of the dogs and my friends up on the wall. You were also allowed to bring flowers into the room, so I had a few plants. Everyone did the best they could to make it feel like home.

The Ward

(Monday, May 13, 2002)

Thanks to Kristen's improving numbers, her nose tube was finally removed on Monday, and she was able to go back to drinking her protein shakes. She was determined not to have any more tubes in her nose, and drank them down with no complaints.

A wonderful surprise arrived from Sully's sister-in-law, Debbie, who was a teacher in New Hampshire. After hearing about Kristen, she'd asked each of the kids in her class to write a letter to Kristen; then, she packaged the letters up and mailed them to us.

I couldn't believe what a kind gesture it was. The letters really lifted Kristen's spirits, and she enjoyed reading every one of them.

* * *

That day, we met a new friend in the ward, a cancer patient who I'll call 'Jeffrey.' Jeffrey was a really great little guy. He was waiting for a bone marrow transplant, which he said was his last chance. Like many of the kids in the ward, he had to live with his condition day by day, with no thoughts about the future. I was amazed at how open he was about his situation, and how—also like many of the kids—he'd somehow managed to come to terms with it.

Of course, all of the parents on 6 North were a mess—the pain and suffering in the ward really leaves its mark on you, especially because kids are involved. Despite all the challenges my own family was facing, I couldn't help but feel guilty, knowing that many of the kids around us had even fewer options, and some might not be around for very long. That kind of thing really hits you hard.

That evening, I visited Jeffrey and we watched a bit of the hockey game. Man, did he ever give me grief about Montreal! We had fun joking about it, but for me, there was a sad edge to the conversation. I mean, try even pretending to get mad at a 13-year-old kid whose last chance for life depends on the bone marrow of a complete stranger, one who may never appear.

Bitter Medicine

(Monday, May 13, to Tuesday, May 14, 2002)

I'm pretty sure that the biggest challenge faced by companies that make medical supplements is to make them taste like, well, something you'd actually want to drink. I'm sure it can't be easy, because some of the things they're hiding in there—like the ingredients that are actually supposed to help you—probably taste awful to begin with.

The protein shake that Kristen had to drink to bring up her weight was a good example. Another one was the phosphate supplement she was given on Monday evening.

Earlier that day, lab tests had shown that Kristen's phosphate levels were too low, so after drinking her protein shake, she was given a supplement that looked like an Alka-Seltzer tablet. It even fizzed up when we added it to a glass of water.

She took a big gulp of it…

…and two minutes later…

…woofed her cookies.

Surely it can't be that bad, I thought.

I dipped the tip of my finger in the drink, touched it to my tongue, and immediately regretted my decision. I was pretty sure I'd have a hard time keeping that stuff down, too.

Despite this minor setback, Kristen felt okay afterwards—although she was a little disappointed that on the first day she was able to drink protein shakes again, she had ended up throwing one up thanks to a fizzy phosphate supplement. She was also worried that they would put the nose tube back in because of this little misadventure. Fortunately, when the fizz finally died down, she was able to finish what was left of the phosphate drink, and her appetite wasn't affected.

* * *

The next morning, we received an update on the lab results. Apparently, Kristen's last phosphate reading had been very different from the previous ones, and so the doctors now suspected that the lab might have misread it; in other words, she may not have needed the phosphate drink after all.

Needless to say, Kristen was less than impressed with this turn of events. Understandable. But I thought back to those six months before she'd been admitted to hospital, when her symptoms had been ignored time and again—and I realized that I'd rather see the doctors err on the side of caution than ignore what might be a serious problem.

Fortunately, that unpleasantness was offset by some really good news: the doctors were very pleased with how Kristen was improving, and told us that if her condition was stable enough, she might be able to leave the hospital in mid-July and wait for the transplant operation at home. We were now used to being cautiously optimistic, but this was still pretty exciting news.

Of course, Kristen would still have to receive her dialysis treatments. The problem was that if they continued her treatments at the hospital, she would still end up travelling back and forth every day, which wouldn't be any better for her than the present situation.

An obvious solution was to set up a dialysis machine in our home. But in order for this to happen, Debbie and I would first have to learn how to run a dialysis session.

The hospital offered to train us. It would be an intensive hands-on course, from 9 to 5 every day, five days a week, over a three-week period.

Although we were excited about finally being able to bring Kristen home, we now also felt a little anxious, and for a few reasons: first, during those three weeks of training, we were told we wouldn't be able to visit Kristen during the day, meaning she would be alone a lot of the time. Second, we were anxious about the training itself: would it cover every possible scenario? And if, heaven forbid, we made a mistake, would we know how to fix it?

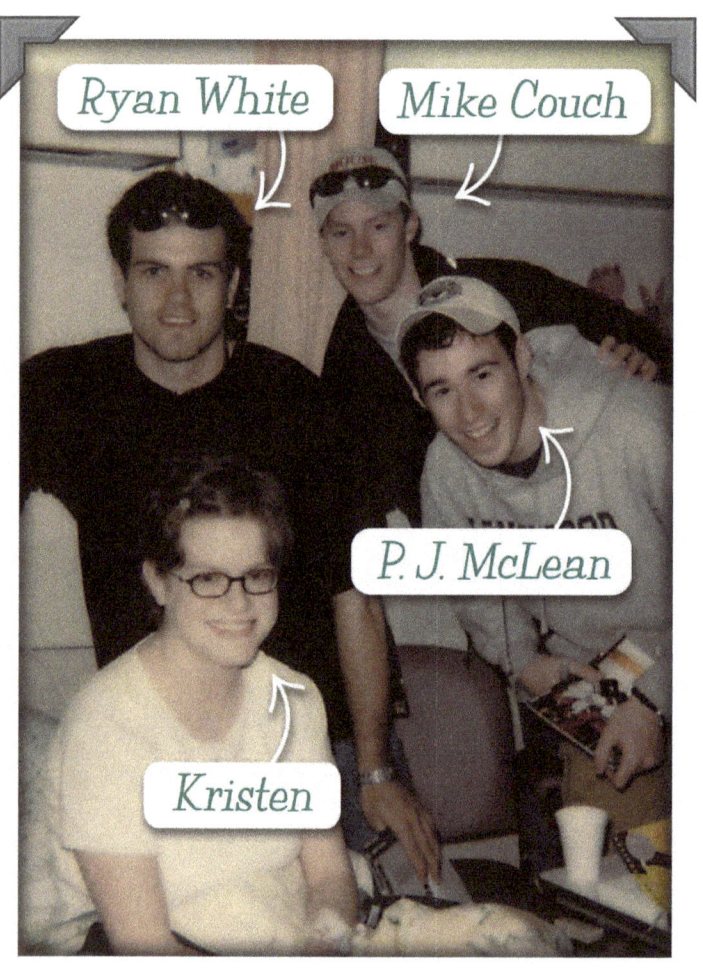

Mooseheads!

(Wednesday, May 15, 2002)

With her numbers continuing to come down, Kristen started the next day in good spirits. And it got even better when some players from our city's Major Junior A hockey team, the Halifax Mooseheads, paid a visit to the ward.

Kristen was thrilled! They actually visited her room, and she got her picture taken with them, complete, of course, with autographs! No doubt she'd be the envy of her friends at school.

KRISTEN REMEMBERS…

I wasn't thrilled at all about the Mooseheads! In fact, Mom chased them down in the hallway despite my fervent disapproval. After all, I was a 15-year-old girl and these were "cute" 18- and 19-year-old boys.

I feigned happiness well…

Later that day, Debbie and I met Jane, the dialysis training coordinator, and we discussed what we'd be learning over the next few weeks. As we discovered, the course would include a lot more than just how to use a dialysis machine. We would also learn how to do everything a nurse has to do to prepare a patient for dialysis, from reading blood test results to giving needles. Although we were intimidated by the range of material that the course would be covering, we quickly warmed to Jane. She was not only knowledgeable, but also very funny and personable, and we looked forward to working with her.

On the scheduling front, Debbie and I were very thankful that Kristen wouldn't be ready to go home for at least another month, so that we would have plenty of time to get up to speed. We were also thankful that we lived so close to the hospital: if we did run into any problems, we were only a few minutes away from expert help.

Meanwhile, I soldiered on with my diet: that day, it would be a western sandwich for breakfast, celery and carrot sticks for snacks, a few cabbage rolls for lunch, and nothing for supper.

Luckily, the day was a busy one, so I had little time to focus on how hungry I was. After our meeting with Jane, I had to rush to a parish council meeting. When that ended a few hours later, I hurried back to the hospital so I could spend some more time with Kristen. By the time I got home that night, I barely had the strength to fall on my pillow.

School Days

(Friday, May 17, 2002)

Because Kristen was first admitted to the hospital shortly after Easter, she ended up missing the last two months of Grade 9. This meant that in addition to being hospitalized, she now also had to worry about how the school administrators would deal with her prolonged absence.

Would they make her repeat the year? If that happened, she'd lose contact with all her classmates as they moved on to Grade 10 and she was forced to repeat Grade 9. Would her teachers give some weight to the fact that she'd already finished three-quarters of the year, and still maintained passing grades in spite of everything that had happened? We all crossed our fingers, knowing that those two months of missed classes would be a huge strike against her.

* * *

Related to that, we were pleasantly surprised to find out that the IWK provided special tutors to help kids keep up with their studies. If Kristen was feeling up to it, we were told the tutors would consult with her school teachers, get the class materials she needed, and help her with her work. There would actually be two people helping her with her studies: one tutor would work with her in English, math, and science, and the other tutor would help her with her French studies.

Although it wasn't the same as being in school, it meant that Kristen at least wouldn't fall too far behind. We also thought it would help keep her mind off the constant anxiety and stress she was having to endure.

KRISTEN REMEMBERS...

When I was going through the tutoring course at the IWK, I really didn't care for it, to be honest. I was always so tired and withdrawn that it took more out of me than it seemed it was worth.

We strive to be our best, and getting straight A's is what we define as being the best. Of course, with my tutors, I was just happy to be sitting up straight and holding a pencil, let alone worrying about my grades. However, the tutorial classes did give me a small sense of normalcy in a world of chaos.

* * *

That week, Kristen received another wonderful surprise from the doctors: because she had been doing so well, after they unhooked her from the machine on Friday, she was allowed to leave the hospital for a few hours to visit her school.

Kristen had really missed her school chums and teachers over the previous month, so she couldn't wait to get there.

Judging from the warm reception she got, they had all missed her, too. It seemed like everyone had questions for her, and she was happy to answer all of them.

The hours passed quickly, and soon it was time to head home. Kristen was actually okay with that: after weeks of being stuck in a hospital bed, she had lost some of her muscle mass, and this meant that even those few hours at her school had left her feeling pretty exhausted. When we got home, she ended up spending her last hour of freedom just resting.

KRISTEN REMEMBERS...
Even after that, during my visits home, I would often just curl up on the couch and fall asleep. I was so sleep deprived when I was in the hospital because I was always poked and prodded and never left alone; when I'd get home, I'd pass right out.

The dogs were thrilled to see her, and cozied up with her as she slept. Of course, an hour isn't very long, and before we knew it, it was time to go back to 6 North.

"One in Twenty"

(Saturday, May 18, to Sunday, May 19, 2002)

On Saturday morning, Kristen, Debbie, and I met with Dr. Crocker to discuss what we needed to do over the coming months to prepare Kristen for the transplant operation. After all the progress we thought we were making, this meeting was quite a reality check.

One statistic he brought up was to do with Kristen's appetite—or lack of it. He warned us that, on average, for every twenty kidney transplants, one patient doesn't make it through surgery. The reason for this is malnutrition. He was very concerned about Kristen being that 'one' because she still hadn't gained enough weight.

Another sobering piece of news was that Kristen had officially been put on the deceased donors waiting list. Although we weren't surprised, we had been dreading this because it meant the selection process would now be completely beyond our control: we would have no idea how long it would take for a donor to become available, or who the donor might be.

Still, what choice did we have? We hadn't yet found a donor among our family and friends, and the hospital had to be prepared for the possibility that we wouldn't.

* * *

On Sunday, we took Kristen home again for another short visit. Four hours isn't very long, and she had just enough time to wash up and rest before having to go back. These trips tired her out, but she was happy to have a few hours away from the ward. Unfortunately, this small taste of freedom would soon create some unexpected drama.

In Isolation

(Monday, May 20, and Tuesday, May 21, 2002)

The next evening was rough. When we brought Kristen home for her four-hour stay, she was feeling really down, and it was her turn to have a brief meltdown.

She was also adamant: she did not want to go back to the hospital.

KRISTEN REMEMBERS…

I was physically and emotionally exhausted. I wanted this nightmare to be over with, so I could return to a degree of teenage normalcy.

I felt terrible for her. And the worse I felt for her, the angrier I became at the circumstances behind her ordeal. As you can imagine, it's hard to be in a positive frame of mind when your child is not only struggling to survive, but also dealing with debilitating depression. To make things worse, her depression, along with the uremia, was killing her appetite, and this was, in turn, bringing down her hemoglobin, to the point where she was now anemic. If her hemoglobin went below 110, she'd have to have an "EPO" needle to bring it up. EPO is short for *epoetin alfa injection*, and it's used to help kidney patients who suffer from anemia. Basically, it triggers your bone marrow to produce more red blood cells.

On top of her general exhaustion, the extra urea in her system was also sapping her energy. Even though the urea level had more or less stabilized, it was still higher than it should be—and we knew it would stay that way until she got a replacement kidney.

Eventually, we managed to convince her to go back to the hospital. Still, we all knew that the next day just held the promise of another four hours of freedom, followed by a return to the place she was starting to see as a prison.

* * *

I spent Tuesday morning working out my frustrations on the links.

When I got home, I found everyone there, including Kristen. After the stress of the previous day, it was nice to hear some good news: Kristen would now be allowed six hours at home, instead of four.

Apparently they were planning to increase the volume of dialysis solution during her exchanges so that they could eventually send her home for 12 hours at a time. That would definitely give her a break from the hospital routine. It would also make the transition easier when she finally moved home in mid-July.

* * *

Later that day, when I took Kristen back to the hospital, they found that she had caught a cold. That's no big deal when everyone around you is healthy, but it's a *really big deal* when you're in a hospital ward.

Kristen was quickly put in isolation in her room. That meant that everyone entering the room had to wash their hands and put on a gown; when they left her room, they had to wash their hands again and put the gown in a special bin.

This was to avoid bringing the germs with them into the rest of the ward; there were so many sick kids on the floor with low immune thresholds that they couldn't afford to catch anything whatsoever. Because it could easily become a life-or-death situation, every single time you left the room, for whatever reason, you had to go through the same routine.

Being healthy and seeing the serious challenges these kids had to face down every single day, it really hit home with me just how fortunate most people are.

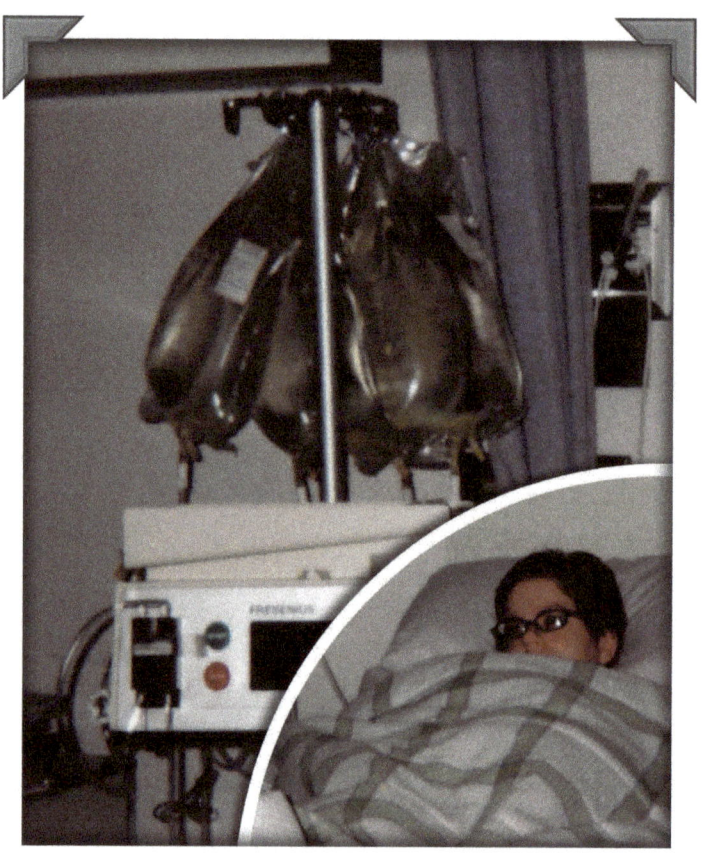

Dialysis kept Kristen alive throughout the summer.

In Training

(Wednesday, May 22, to Friday, May 24, 2002)

On Wednesday, Debbie and I began our dialysis training. We were excited about starting the course, but still worried about being away from Kristen for so much of the next three weeks. All we could do was promise ourselves that we would visit her at every opportunity.

KRISTEN REMEMBERS…

My parents had to learn how to work the dialysis machine because it would be my lifeline throughout the summer.

Over the next few days, the learning curve was pretty steep: The first things we learned about were Kristen's medications and how to give her an EPO needle. Once Kristen returned home, we would be responsible for keeping an eye on her hemoglobin level, and giving her an EPO shot if it fell too low.

Along with that, we learned how to read blood test results so that we could monitor Kristen's condition from day to day. We also learned more basic skills, like how to take a temperature, listen for a heartbeat with a stethoscope, and take a pulse reading. It was a little nerve-wracking to know that everything we were now learning would soon be necessary to ensure our daughter's survival. To help relieve our anxiety, Jane would often lighten the mood of our "classes" with much-needed humour, and these moments of laughter really helped to ground us!

By the end of the week, Kristen had recovered from her cold, which meant she could go back to taking brief 'vacations' away from the hospital. She was also beginning to accept the fact that she would have to go back each day when the time was up. I suspected that it would be easier for her because she was now off dialysis for about eight hours each day, which meant that her visits home would be less rushed.

Meanwhile, Gary was starting to look like a match, with all the tests indicating he was a good candidate. Of course, they still wanted to run preliminary tests on anyone else who contacted the transplant coordinator, just in case there was a better match. By 'better,' I mean that if Gary was okay in, say, four out of six tests, that might be enough for a match. But if someone else was okay in five out of six tests, then they would go with that person instead. We were told that the hospital would have a pretty good idea of the best match by early the following week.

We also learned that if Kristen were an adult, and we knew that Gary was the best match, they would already have been confirming a transplant date. Apparently, adult patients are processed more quickly than children, and once they find a match, the transplant operation and release from hospital happen in pretty rapid succession.

But at the IWK, they were less concerned with speed than with ensuring that each patient was in the best possible shape prior to the transplant, and also that the donor's kidney was the best one for that patient. In Kristen's case, they wouldn't even consider setting a date until her weight was up. We were also told that once the transplant was complete, they would make sure Kristen was fully recovered before being released.

This approach was obviously effective, given their 96-percent success rate!

Wake-Up Call

(Monday, May 27, 2002)

On Monday, we met with the transplant coordinator. She confirmed that Gary was the best match out of all the volunteers, which meant they would now proceed to more advanced tests. I couldn't believe how positive this (well, 30-year-old) kid was. He joked that all he was worried about was what the 'shrink' was going to find in their interview. Funny how common that fear is.

We also received some news that really put the whole situation into perspective: we were told that when we'd first brought Kristen in a month earlier, she was literally within days of collapse and death. The doctors confirmed that if she hadn't seen her cardiologist when she had, he wouldn't have noticed her enlarged heart, and Kristen would now probably be dead.

Once again, I felt that familiar chill down my back, as I thought how fortunate we were that her appointments happened to be so close together.

* * *

Due to Kristen's low body-weight, and the ongoing selection process, we were told that the earliest possible time for a transplant would be the end of July. Assuming that Kristen would be allowed to go home in mid-June, that meant Debbie and I would be responsible for her dialysis and daily care for at least a couple of weeks.

With this in mind, we forged ahead with our training. That day, we learned how to take blood pressure, which I actually found kind of interesting. You start by putting an inflatable cuff around the patient's upper arm and pumping it with air. Then, you hold a stethoscope against the inside crook of their arm (where it bends). You slowly release the air and listen for a series of pulse beats. The first "thump" in the series tells you when their heart is fully contracted and pumping out blood—that's their *systolic* (highest) pressure. The last "thump" tells you when their heart is relaxed and refilling with blood—that's their *diastolic* (lowest) pressure.

I always had a hard time finding them, but Debbie, even with her hearing loss, was able to catch Kristen's beats perfectly.

* * *

In the afternoon, another package arrived: a handmade book of poems created by a class-full of kids in New Hampshire! Sully's sister-in-law Debbie wanted to let Kristen know they were thinking about her. It was a really thoughtful gift, and helped to lift Kristen's spirits during what had been a particularly bad week.

Home Away from Home

(Sunday, June 9, 2002)

By the second week in June, Danielle and Allison had finished their exams and were waiting for their final marks. We all crossed our fingers for Danielle. In fact, Debbie and I promised ourselves we would enjoy a celebratory bottle of wine if she passed. We would know one way or another by the following Friday.

Kristen was now able to come home for 11 hours at a time. She really enjoyed being away from the hospital, although every so often, she would get depressed and want to go back early. We suspected her numbers were to blame. Despite the dialysis treatments, her creatinine had once again climbed to around 1000; her phosphate was also above normal, which caused her to feel weak and tired a lot of the time.

KRISTEN REMEMBERS:

I loved to be home, but I also enjoyed being at the hospital. I was getting to know the nurses on a more personal level, and after six weeks of being a patient, I was also getting very used to hospital life. Each day was a series of timed events, and I had a very predictable schedule for dialysis, medication, and so on.

I didn't like being home in the summer because my friends were asking me to go out and have fun with them, but I needed to be hooked up to a machine at a certain time. That sense of normalcy was taken away from me and I didn't feel like I belonged in my circle of friends anymore because I had this large thing looming over my head.

When I was at the hospital, I was the "star student" because my condition was "normal" for what I was going through and I was "healthy" for what I was going through. I felt like I fit in more with my peers at the hospital than I did with my friends when I was home.

Meanwhile, Debbie and I were gearing up for our final week of training. The previous week, we'd learned how to put on a shower dressing and a sterile dressing, and how to give someone a needle. (I was actually starting to notice how handy this training was: A few days earlier, while carrying a heavy box of dialysis solution into the basement, I'd tripped on the steps. I scraped up my knee pretty badly, and my mind automatically focused on how I would apply a dressing using bandages and tape, if they'd actually been handy. Move over, George Clooney!)

That week, we would start training with an actual dialysis machine. It was a little intimidating, but we felt pretty confident that we would be ready when Kristen finally came home.

At the same time, some of the hospital staff were now on vacation, so Gary's tests were put on hold until the lab people came back. There was no question that the staff had earned their time off (and then some), but because we were sitting on pins and needles waiting for test results, I have to admit I was counting the days until their vacation time was over!

Some Sad News; Another Crisis

(Monday, June 10, to Wednesday, June 12, 2002)

On Monday, there was a very sad occurrence in the ward. Some of the kids were cancer patients, and we lost one of them that day: a dear little girl. She couldn't have been any more than two years old. Although the nurses wouldn't talk (and rightly so), I had found out about it from another parent. We all felt devastated.

At times like that, it seems that life isn't right. And although I know God has a plan, I'll still be wanting an explanation for a few things when I get to Heaven.

* * *

Two days later, we were dealing with a new crisis of our own. Over the previous week, Kristen's calcium, phosphate, and urea numbers had mysteriously begun to climb again. This had brought back her nausea, fatigue, and other symptoms, which in turn sent her back into a depression.

Even though the doctors weren't sure why this was happening, her climbing numbers didn't seem to alarm them too much. In my mind, though, this was a step backward, not forward, and I knew that Kristen would see it as another stumbling block that separated her from her home, her friends, and all those other things most of us take for granted.

KRISTEN REMEMBERS...

My attitude toward my friendships had begun to change. My life was spiralling out of control, so my friends' materialistic concerns and minor complaints (teenager-based things—well, normal teenager things) now irritated me because I felt sort of jealous that they were living a normal life. I was starting to disconnect from that part of my life.

One thing that kept us going was that Gary's test results had all been positive so far. Of course, thanks to our experiences up to that point, I didn't dare take anything for granted until we had a confirmed date for the transplant. I did know that we would be indebted to Gary forever for what he was about to do.

Late Wednesday morning, they unhooked Kristen, and I took her home before Debbie and I began our afternoon training session. By this point, we knew how to set up the dialysis machine, and how to run through all the computer screens to complete a treatment. Although it was pretty straightforward, I now appreciated having a full three weeks to not just learn the basics, but also practice and understand the entire process.

The Award Goes To...

(Wednesday, June 12, to Thursday, June 13, 2002)

Late Wednesday afternoon, I received a call from Sacred Heart School. Because Kristen's marks up to Easter had still been above average, they decided to extrapolate her grades so that she could pass! We were grateful for their decision.

That wasn't all, though. I was told that Kristen would be receiving a special award at the Grade 9 graduation ceremony the following day.

KRISTEN REMEMBERS:

The Anita Thomas Memorial Award was given to students who, despite great adversity, were able to persevere and accomplish their goals, while also maintaining a positive attitude.

The problem was that we didn't know if Kristen would feel well enough to attend the ceremony. To add to the challenge, they wanted the special award to be a surprise, so if she wasn't feeling 100 percent, we would somehow have to motivate her to go. (Of course, we decided that we'd tell her the truth if we absolutely had to.)

During the call, I couldn't help but ask about Danielle. That brought even more good news: she'd passed Grade 7—what a relief. Apparently she was 1.1 points short of the passing grade of 60, but they also took into consideration what our family had gone through that spring.

Later, I would find out that Allison had passed Grade 5, and with flying colours! This meant we were "three for three" (with "two-for-two" very proud parents).

* * *

The next day, we were very relieved that Kristen felt well enough to attend the ceremony. When we got there, we were touched to learn that many of Kristen's teachers and fellow students were looking forward to her being there to celebrate with them.

As with most graduation ceremonies, they conferred the special awards first, followed by the graduation certificates. I knew that Kristen was looking forward to receiving her diploma, but she was completely surprised when she was called up early in the proceedings to receive the Anita Thomas Award.

We were so proud as Kristen walked across the stage to accept it. The award seemed like a confirmation from her teachers and fellow students, that she'd succeeded in spite of enormous challenges, and that they were also very proud of her for doing so.

Needless to say, there weren't too many dry eyes in the school auditorium that afternoon.

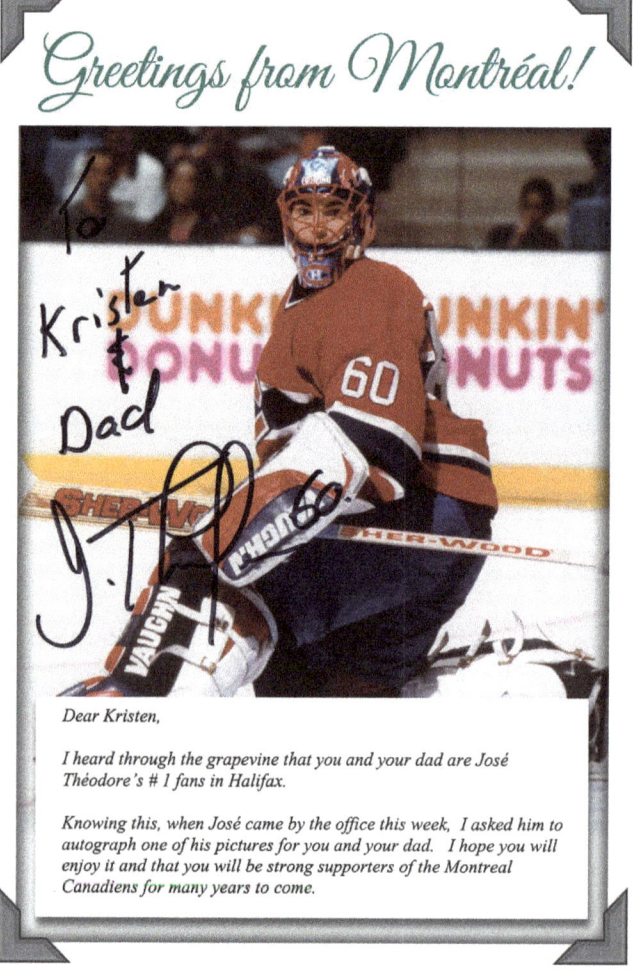

Dear Kristen,

I heard through the grapevine that you and your dad are José Théodore's #1 fans in Halifax.

Knowing this, when José came by the office this week, I asked him to autograph one of his pictures for you and your dad. I hope you will enjoy it and that you will be strong supporters of the Montreal Canadiens for many years to come.

Special Delivery

(Thursday afternoon, June 13, 2002)

After returning home from the graduation ceremony, we noticed an oversized envelope in our mailbox. I checked the return address and was surprised to see it was from the head office of the Montreal Canadiens hockey team. I carefully opened the package, reached in, and pulled out a letter along with a picture of their star goalie, José Théodore.

The letter was from Pierre Boivin, the president of the Montreal Canadiens. He said he understood that Kristen and I were avid Montreal fans, and thought we'd enjoy having a signed picture of José. I looked at the picture again and, sure enough, it was signed to Kristen and me.

What a thrill! Of course, I then thought, "Why would he send this to us? He doesn't even know me."

After a moment, it clicked in: Back when Sully was working for Nike, Pierre Boivin was the president of the company. Later, when Pierre moved on from Nike, he was hired by the Montreal Canadiens. That had to be the connection.

I emailed Sully about it and he confirmed what I had guessed.

Sully knew that I was a huge Canadiens fan. Unbeknownst to me, he'd called up his old boss, told him about Kristen, and asked if Pierre could do something special for her. José Théodore happened to be in his office while they were on the phone, and so Pierre got José to sign the picture. Then he put the letter together and sent it off.

Kristen didn't have a clue who either José or Pierre were, but I, being a faithful Canadiens fan, was excited enough for both of us. I went around the ward showing the letter to everyone.

Of course, considering what would happen the following day, this would turn out to be a much-needed morale boost.

Another Man Down

(Tuesday, June 18, 2002)

One of our worst days started off pretty quietly. Midway through our training session, we stopped for a coffee break, and so Debbie and I decided to head up to the sixth floor and spend some time with Kristen.

Just after we arrived, Gary came into the room. He looked pretty downcast, and I immediately got a cold feeling in my stomach. He told us that his latest test, a urinalysis, showed there was a problem.

Up to then, everything had seemed fine. His blood work and tissue count both looked good, and we really had our hopes up.

But the urinalysis results had shown excess protein in his system; this was a sign that Gary was having trouble processing waste. It turned out he had been using a high-protein drink for weight-training and it was overflowing into his urine, a sign that he may have damaged his kidneys. They'd told Gary he would have to wait several months to ensure his body was clear of the high-protein drink before they would test him again.

We were devastated. We had been let down before, but this time we'd felt positive that we finally had a donor. Once more, it seemed like the carpet was being pulled out from under us. Up to that point, we'd been thinking that, after all the other setbacks, at least we'd finally levelled out, and there was nowhere to go but up (or at worst, sideways). Now, we'd found that there was still someplace even lower.

Gary felt so awful about the results; he'd really wanted to help. Looking back, I'm still not sure who I felt worse for at that moment: Debbie, Kristen, or him.

Later that day, Sully wrote to say how disappointed and upset they all were, and that his family were all praying that someone else would be found. He ended by saying, "Our thoughts are with you guys. Something good will come out of this."

Although I appreciated his words and prayers, at the time, it still felt like a big void had opened up in front of us. If something good was waiting on the horizon, I couldn't see it from where I was standing.

Back to Square One

(Friday, June 21, 2002)

Now that Gary had been taken off the list—at least for the next several months—it meant that we were back to square one. This also meant they would have to fast-track Kristen on the deceased donors waiting list. We were told that children on the list are already considered first, but Kristen's serious condition meant she would be bumped up. That was good news, but it still didn't guarantee that she would receive a kidney in time.

KRISTEN REMEMBERS...

They told Gary he needed to stop using the protein drink and come back in six months. Did I have six months? Certainly the dialysis had kept me alive, but how long could I last?

They also began to call up other people who had contacted the transplant coordinator to donate—including Richard and Judy and our friend Cliff—and asked them to come in for blood work. It would be yet another week before we knew these results.

Regardless, I was thankful they had come forward as volunteers. It offered us some hope in an otherwise grim situation.

I was also cheered up by another development. Over the previous six weeks, along with dieting and exercising, I had been begging the doctors for another chance to be tested. Now it looked like my efforts had finally paid off, because I was told I would soon be given another 24-hour blood pressure test. They said it was to make sure that the earlier results were accurate. Whatever the reason was, I didn't care. All that mattered was that I had another chance to get back on the train!

Now I would find out whether my exercising and dieting over the previous six weeks had made a difference. Would my blood pressure still be too high? Had I lost enough weight? Like the other volunteers, I wouldn't find out anything for at least a week.

PART IV

Try Again!

Thinking Positive

Oddly enough, what I'd come to think of as my diet and exercise routine hadn't really started that way.

On that morning six weeks earlier, when I'd decided to leave the car at home and walk to the hospital, I hadn't consciously thought, "Well, let's start working off those pounds!"

In the back of my mind, I guess I thought it might be helpful to do some walking, but I had no real goal in mind.

At that time, I had been on my new diet for about a week, and I was really struggling with it. My intake of calories was a lot lower than normal, and so I wasn't exactly a bundle of energy; a new exercise regimen wouldn't have been at the top of my To-Do list.

So, on that chilly morning back in May, it had really just been me going for a walk.

But a funny thing happened the next day: the first walk hadn't been so terrible, so I made the journey again.

And then again on the third day.

Soon, it had become a regular part of my daily schedule, and on some days I was even walking both to and from the hospital.

This wasn't the first time I'd made an effort to lose weight, but I had to look back an awfully long time to remember when it had happened before. How long before? Well, would you believe junior high school?

One year, all my buddies went out to join a minor league football team, so, not wanting to be left out, I decided to join the team along with them. The problem was that I needed to lose a few pounds because of a weight restriction. I had a month before tryouts began, so every morning, I would get up early and run around the block before school. I absolutely hated every step, but I was determined to make the cut!

When the big day finally arrived, I stood on the scale—and was promptly hoisted up by a fellow player who'd snuck up behind me and lifted me by my pants! For a few seconds, instead of just meeting the requirement, I actually weighed in about twenty pounds less. Fortunately, after he set me down, I still managed to weigh in below the requirement, and I was able to play ball.

Now, decades later, I faced another challenge based on my weight, and I was confronting it the same way. But a lot of years had gone by since my junior high football days, and I had to wonder, would all my efforts now make any difference?

I'd find out soon enough.

Second Chance

(Wednesday, July 3, to Thursday, July 4, 2002)

The first Wednesday in July, they strapped a blood pressure cuff on my arm for a second time.

It had been almost two months since my first test, and I felt I'd come a long way since then, both physically and psychologically. And, thanks to my recent dialysis training, I already had a pretty good idea of how this new test might turn out.

As part of our home dialysis training, Debbie and I started every day by checking each other's temperature, pulse, and blood pressure. Since mid-May, when we started, I had seen my blood pressure slowly dropping, and according to the calibrated scale we had set up for Kristen, I was now down to 240 pounds; I'd actually lost 20 pounds since visiting my doctor in late April! All of this was thanks to my diet and daily walks.

That day, we were finally given Kristen's release date. If her condition remained stable, we would be able to bring her home the following Wednesday. In the meantime, until she went home, Kristen was moved to a room down the hall from the nurses' station.

KRISTEN REMEMBERS...
I was moved there so that when my dialysis machine's alarm went off, Mom and Dad would be given time to fix the problem before the nurses arrived.

On Wednesday night, I stayed in the hospital with Kristen to troubleshoot the dialysis machine. Everything went okay—just two alarms went off, and both were easy to fix.

* * *

On Thursday, I dropped off the blood pressure monitor at the hospital. Although I was pretty sure the results would be within the required range, I couldn't help feeling jittery, because there was so much riding on them.

Fortunately, I didn't need to worry: when I finally got the call, I was told that my blood pressure was in the normal range. That meant I was back on the donor train! At the time, I remember joking with Kristen that she could end up being a Montreal fan, because she might be using a kidney that had belonged to one.

KRISTEN REMEMBERS...

I was never a born-again Montreal fan. However, I will cheer for them over any other team in the playoffs.

Now the serious testing would begin. I was given urine bottles to take home, and I was scheduled for major blood work on the following Monday.

* * *

On Thursday night, it was Debbie's turn to stay with Kristen and watch the dialysis machine. We all crossed our fingers, hoping for the same results that I'd had on Thursday.

Silent Alarms

(Friday, July 5, 2002)

The next morning, Debbie phoned me from the hospital. She said she was happy to report that Kristen had slept through the entire night, without any alarms.

Well…

When I got to the hospital, Kristen admitted to us that there were alarms, but that she'd managed to fix them. She felt good about this because it meant she could troubleshoot the system herself if necessary.

Debbie wasn't quite as happy, though. She was now worried that she might not hear the alarms when Kristen was back at home—especially when I had to travel to North Carolina for a week in mid-July. I wasn't too worried, though, knowing that we still had a month to practice before I left.

* * *

Later that morning, Kristen's calcium level started to rise. Seeing this, the doctors decided to give her a calcium supplement to return it to normal. Although the odds of Kristen having an adverse reaction were low, we were warned about one possible side effect that was pretty scary…

KRISTEN REMEMBERS…

I was told that when the calcium was administered, there was a 1 in 14 chance that I could go into shock and lose my ability to breathe. It was petrifying because up to this point, with everything that had happened, I always seemed to be that "one"!

The nurses were ready with oxygen as they slowly put the solution into my IV, so, of course, although I was scared, I had faith that the nurses would protect me. THANKFULLY nothing happened.

Despite the risk, the treatment was worth it, because it made her feel better and brought back her appetite. We were also told that this development wouldn't affect Kristen's schedule; she would still be able to go home the following Wednesday.

* * *

That afternoon, I took home a bunch of urine sample bottles, which I spent the weekend filling at regular intervals. On Monday, I dropped the samples off at the IWK and then had 12 vials of blood taken. After that, all those bottles and vials were sent to the lab.

Now it was a matter of waiting for the test results. I was told it would take about a week.

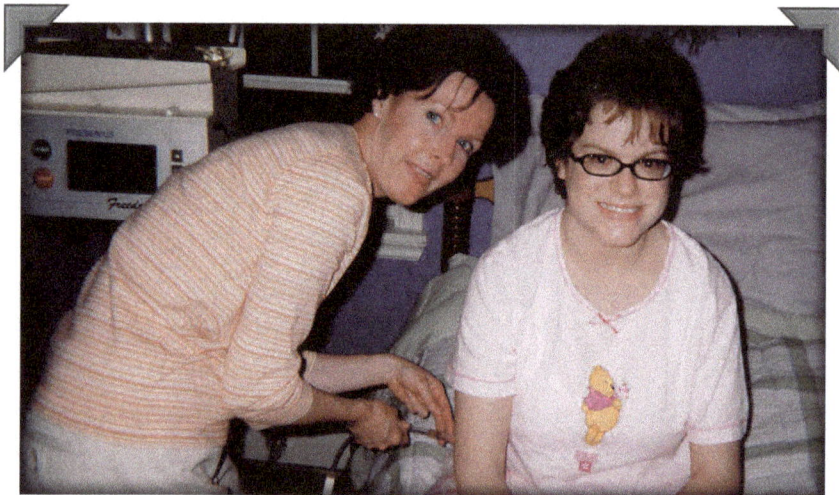

Running a home dialysis session.

Finally Home

(Wednesday, July 10, 2002)

As promised, we were able to take Kristen home on Wednesday. Everyone was excited for her—doctors and nurses included.

That day, Debbie and I received a certificate—with "honours"—showing that we had completed our home dialysis training. (We eventually framed it and put it in Kristen's room.) Debbie presented the floor with one of her beautiful tole paintings (which they hung up in the family room), and we gave the staff one of my famous (in my mind only) orange-chocolate cheese cakes—which was gone in half an hour.

* * *

Before we left the hospital, I got a call at the nurses' station from the transplant co-ordinator. She told me the results were positive for my blood work and urinalysis, which meant I could move on to the cardiogram on Thursday. It was a perfect way to cap an already great morning.

After that, Kristen was unhooked from her monitors, and we left the sixth floor.

During the drive home—as Kristen sat in the front seat and Debbie rested in the back—an innocent bit of conversation brought up another "moment." I mentioned to Kristen that I didn't know whether I was happier about the positive test results or about her coming home. When Debbie heard this, she began to cry with joy—basically, Niagara Falls was happening in the back seat.

KRISTEN REMEMBERS...

I remember Mom crying in the back seat and Dad saying, "There she goes again," jokingly, of course. It was just a combination of emotions and exhaustion.

Things were finally starting to work out. After so many weeks of close calls and emergency treatments, the constant worry and countless reversals—this was our ray of sun, this was our sunrise.

Kristen's return home was also a special milestone to us: with her condition now stable, and our home dialysis training finished, we considered this the end of phase one. The second phase would now begin in earnest, as we focused on and prepared for the transplant operation.

Timing

(Tuesday, July 16, 2002)

After Kristen came home, our lives began to settle into something resembling normal. Of course, if we needed a reality check, all we had to do was look in the basement, where all of her dialysis supplies were now stored. The day after we'd brought her home, six weeks' worth of materials and supplies had been delivered to our house, with the dialysate alone filling up 90 boxes.

In the meantime, we carried on with our lives.

On Tuesday morning, Debbie took Allison to the doctor to get tested for allergies. Because I had scheduled some time on the links, we had asked Debbie's niece, Cheryl, to come over and stay with the kids that day.

As luck would have it, Cheryl had called the previous night to tell us her car had broken down and she wouldn't be able to come over. This meant golf was out, because only Debbie and I could oversee Kristen's disconnection from the machine. Needless to say, as I looked at the beautiful weather outside, my mood was anything but.

KRISTEN REMEMBERS...

I'm always giving Dad grief about golfing, and I had to laugh because he was sooooo cranky that day for missing golf.

Because I was home, I went with Kristen and Debbie to the hospital that afternoon when Kristen got her blood work done. While we were there, I received word that the transplant coordinator wanted to see me. In fact, she had been trying to call us at home, and was paging us all over 6 North. She'd also left a message that she had more stuff for me to pick up—I assumed it was requisitions for more testing.

When we finally caught up with her, she told us some news that made up for all the setbacks we'd gone through over the previous month: I was a 100-percent match with Kristen!

KRISTEN REMEMBERS...

After Dad found out the good news about being a match, he felt bad for having been so ticked off. Men and their golf—I will never understand their passion for such a yawn-worthy sport. (Sorry, Daddy.)

The coordinator hadn't seen a match like this in a long time. In fact, she said it was very rare for results to be this perfect, where everything matched, right across the board. She joked that Debbie and I had mixed up our genes and put them into Kristen perfectly! I suspected that the Big Guy Upstairs may have played a part in us getting those results.

Now that I was officially compatible, I was scheduled to meet with a few different specialists. The blood work would also get a little more involved now, with tests for things like HIV and other communicable diseases. I would also need to fill in a very detailed questionnaire that would tell them everything they needed to know about me.

Still, I was so relieved about the results that I didn't care what hoops I now needed to jump through. I had never wanted this to go any further than me for a lot of reasons. One was that it was my duty as a father to do anything I could for my kids. Another reason was that I really didn't want anyone else—including Gary—to be affected. Now, the responsibility would rest on my shoulders, and it was a weight I felt comfortable with.

Fountain of Generosity

(Tuesday, July 23, 2002)

The following week, I went for another round of tests at the IWK. It started with an ultrasound. To get the clearest picture, they wanted my bladder to be as large as it could be, so I had been told to drink about four glasses of water before coming in that morning. Being the cautious type, I decided to drink more than double that amount, figuring that if four glasses of water would give them a good 35mm picture, nine glasses would give them a fantastic IMAX picture, in 3D.

Of course, I hadn't really considered that all that fluid would eventually start looking for an exit, and not necessarily at a time of my choosing.

For the ultrasound test, they injected a special fluid using an IV; it felt warm going in, which was actually kind of nice (although probably not the best sensation for a guy who was already needing to go to the bathroom). Apparently this fluid would make it easier for them to check how well my urinary tract was working.

Another reason for the procedure was to confirm that I actually had an extra kidney to donate. That surprised me, but I was told that about 1 in 750 people are actually born with only one kidney.

As it turned out, everything was a "go" on both counts: my bladder was working fine, and I had two kidneys.

After that, I went to have more blood taken, this time for tests that looked for HIV, Hep A, Hep C, and so on. Although we weren't expecting any surprises there, they had to be sure.

Unfortunately, I had to wait a while for all these tests, because a lot of other people were also lined up in front of me to get their blood work done. Afterwards, I needed to pee (big surprise), so I went searching for a washroom, even though, in about 20 minutes, I would be meeting with the nephrologist, and I would also need to pee for him. Of course, having drunk about 70 ounces of water that morning, I was sure I could comply in every instance.

The nephrologist—a nice fellow named Dr. Panek—asked me a lot of questions, and then gave me a physical exam to check my weight, blood pressure, heart rate, and so on. After that, we went over all the pros and cons, for Kristen and myself, of the upcoming operation.

One important thing I learned was how a kidney transplant improves the recipient's quality of life, by getting them off of dialysis. I had assumed that dialysis was a miracle treatment that you could be on indefinitely, but that's not the case. In fact, if you're on dialysis treatment for too long, you're bound to run into problems. One major complication is weight gain: dialysate solution contains dextrose—a type of sugar—and so you can end up absorbing hundreds of extra calories from it every day, which leads to you packing on extra pounds. Worse, if you're diabetic, absorbing all that dextrose can also lead to high blood sugar.

Over time, continuous dialysis treatment can also result in you getting a hernia. This is because your stomach muscles have to hold all that dialysis fluid in your abdomen for several hours during every dwell time. This constant strain can lead to a bulge wherever your abdominal wall is weak—so, you might develop a hernia in your groin, at the spot where the catheter comes out of your body, or even in your belly button (making your *innie* an *outie*).

Another thing I didn't know was that, over time (usually a matter of years), peritoneal dialysis gets less and less effective; in fact, at a certain point, if you don't get a transplant, you may have to switch over to hemodialysis—which, of course, brings its own set of challenges and problems.

So, for all these reasons, a patient's quality of life definitely improves once they have a new kidney and they're able to leave dialysis behind.

For the donor, I learned that the benefits are mostly psychological, but they are profound. You get the personal satisfaction of knowing that you made a huge difference in someone else's life—ten-fold if it's someone you care about (a big motivator in my case). On top of that, your self-esteem can also get a tremendous boost. (This made sense: since being approved, I generally felt more positive and full of energy.)

When we were finished, he said, "I'm going to recommend that you be the donor."

Yes! I thought, *Finally!*

Then he added, "But first, you have to talk to the psychiatrist."

I walked out of his office, thinking I might actually *need* a shrink, because this drawn-out selection process was probably going to drive me crazy.

* * *

Assuming the meeting with the psychiatrist went well, the scheduling would now be in the hands of the coordinator, whose job it was to confirm that an operating room would be available at the hospital on the day they needed it. At that point, they were looking at some time in late August.

Meanwhile, Kristen was having her good and bad days, as all teenagers will. I thought that in some ways, she was dealing with the situation much better than Debbie and me; but I also thought this might be from the uncanny way teenagers sometimes have of not realizing the full extent of what's happening around them. Maybe that's what maturity and hard experience bring: a clearer view of how difficult every roadblock in front of you is going to be. Of course, I sometimes wonder if this knowledge isn't overrated.

Meeting the Shrink

(Friday, August 3, to Monday, August 5, 2002)

I finished the first Friday in August with a trip to a psychiatrist's office (something that many people probably feel like doing by the time Friday rolls around). In my case, it was to see if I was mentally prepared to be a donor. Dr. Stokes spoke with me for quite a while, and we covered a lot of territory.

One of the questions that really struck me was whether I had put any thought into what life would be like after the operation. Having spent the previous few months wondering when—or even whether—my daughter would find a donor, I hadn't even bothered to think past the transplant. Having never gone through such a frightening, life-altering experience before, I had only been able to cope this far by living day to day. It hadn't occurred to me to think that far into the future.

In a way, this whole exercise felt kind of pointless to me. After all, it wasn't like there was any real choice here. Play all the what-if games and run all the psychological evaluations you want; where your loved ones are concerned, you do what you have to do to help them. You have to live with your choices, and for most people, no amount of rationalizing could justify a selfish decision at a time like this. I'm pretty sure that, when faced with a similar situation, most people would feel the same way I do.

As I told Dr. Stokes, there were only two things I wanted to know when I woke up after the operation. The first—how Kristen was doing—made sense to him. The second—what day it was—required an explanation. I guess it goes to show you the funny directions your mind can take when you give it free rein: I was so afraid something would go wrong and that I would wake up days, months, or even years down the road. I had never been in the hospital for any kind of operation before, and so I had no idea what to expect; unfortunately, my overactive imagination was more than willing to fill in the blanks with worst-case scenarios.

* * *

Meanwhile, life continued. That weekend, I had to prepare for my trip to Raleigh, where I would be attending an important convention. Despite it being so close to the operation date, I had no choice but to attend, as I was being installed as the incoming president of the Honorable Order of the Blue Goose, an international organization of people who work in the insurance industry.

I would be gone for most of the week, returning on the following Monday. Thankfully, Debbie was now a lot more comfortable running the dialysis machine, and knew how to deal with any problems that might arise. I can remember one thing that seemed to set it off: when the tube became kinked, it shut off the flow of dialysis solution into Kristen's stomach. Fortunately, all Kristen had to do was roll over to undo the kink; then we pressed a certain button on the machine, and everything went back to working properly.

The day before I left, we received some great news: the transplant date had finally been set, for Monday, August 28.

Raleigh and Back

(Tuesday, August 13, to Monday, August 19, 2002)

I left for Raleigh the following Tuesday. Although it was a big thrill for me to be installed as the president of the Blue Goose organization, my excitement was—not surprisingly—overshadowed by the drama at home. The outpouring of concern and support from the other members was a bit overwhelming to me. Whenever I talked to people, I felt surrounded by genuine warmth and caring, and I received many hugs and good wishes for a successful outcome.

At the same time, I hadn't been able to shake an irrational fear that had been bugging me for weeks: I had a weird premonition that something would happen to me—perhaps during the convention or even on the flight to or from Raleigh—and that I would end up leaving my wife and daughter both on their own and back at square one. Of course, it was just my imagination running through the worst possible scenarios, but it didn't matter. It still felt real, and was probably made a lot worse because I was keeping all my thoughts bottled up to avoid making anyone around me feel anxious.

Still, throughout the convention, I put on a brave face and focused on my exercise regimen and diet. Around 5 a.m. every morning, I would climb out of bed, head down to the exercise room as soon as it opened, and spend a half-hour on the treadmill—something I would never have considered doing before. Then I'd head back up to my room to get ready for the day. During meals, I also received a lot of help from people who made sure I kept to my diet.

In my acceptance speech, I poked fun at myself by pointing out that my presidency would be an historic one: it would surely be the first time an incoming president began his reign recuperating in a bed in a children's hospital!

* * *

In spite of all my worries, the trip ended up going very well, and I returned from Raleigh the following Monday, tired but happy to be home. The weather that greeted me couldn't have been nicer—hot and dry, and totally unique to our part of the world at that time of year.

That day, the doctors gave me some information about the upcoming surgery, including which of my kidneys they would be using: they had decided to harvest the right kidney. Apparently, that was because it had one less artery and that artery was very long, so they would have a lot of tissue to connect with.

Of course, this meant that during my recovery, I would only be able to sleep on my left side until I was disconnected from all the tubes.

Hearing all of these details really drove home the fact that soon, I would be lying on an operating table, and having part of my insides removed by these guys. I knew they were the best in their field, but it still gave me a chill.

I was cheered up later that afternoon by an email from Sully: Kate, their daughter, was back from camp, and couldn't wait to go back next year; Maureen was doing well, recovering from a recent surgery; and they'd both had a wonderful time at a recent house party hosted by some mutual friends—and, of course, everyone wished that Debbie and I had been there.

Reading this message from my old buddy, I once again thought how lucky we were to have such good people in our lives. During our more difficult moments, it was these well-wishes and thoughtful messages that helped us feel a little more connected to the "real" world.

PART V

The Big Day

Final Tests

(Late August, 2002)

Over the next two weeks, we looked after Kristen at home, only taking her into the hospital for blood tests and checkups. With the Raleigh trip over, I felt a sense of relief, knowing that Debbie and I were once again both watching over Kristen. At the same time, the upcoming operation was beginning to consume a lot of my thoughts.

It would also throw a monkey wrench into my regular fall schedule. My involvement with the upcoming football season at Saint Mary's University was one example. (I was actually the announcer for both football and hockey, a job I hold to this day.) I was worried that I might end up missing the start of the season, and would have to find someone else to fill in for me.

And then, of course, there was my golf schedule.

With the big day approaching, I was planning to sneak in a few extra rounds, and had already booked tee times with a couple of golfing buddies over the following week. Unfortunately, my golf obsession led to some friction with one of the surgeons.

I had to book an early tee time one morning because I was scheduled to meet with the surgeon that afternoon. It was obvious the guy wasn't a golfer because when the transplant nurse was arranging my appointment and I told them I played golf that day, the surgeon just gave me a look that said, "Too bad."

I know that many readers will now be shrugging and saying, "Yeah, too bad." It reminds me of something funny that Sully once told me: One day, his nephew came home from a baseball game and told the family that he'd just thrown a no-hitter. When his mother heard this, she smiled sympathetically and said, "Don't worry, dear. You'll have better luck next time."

Your response to what she said will depend on how familiar you are with baseball: if it made you smile, then you're probably a sports fan, and you might also have some sympathy for my predicament!

* * *

Because neither Kristen nor I had experienced any complications or problems, we were now given an updated schedule.

Although the 28th was the big day, Kristen would actually be checking into the IWK on the 24th so that she could see the heart doctor and other specialists. (I would check in on the 27th, the day before the operation.)

On the 26th, we were both scheduled for more blood tests. In Kristen's case, it was to make sure she hadn't developed any more antibodies. We weren't too worried because that would only happen if Kristen had recently had a blood transfusion. She'd only had two in April, and none since then.

One major concern for me was Debbie, who was suddenly going to have a lot on her plate while both Kristen and I were in the hospital. Debbie would now have to look after Allison and Danielle (and also help them prepare for the upcoming school year), in addition to spending whatever free time she had visiting us at the hospital.

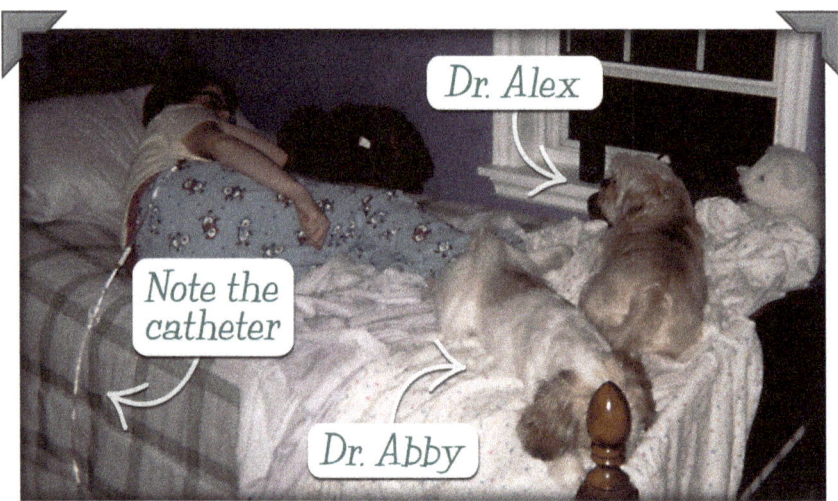

Three's company!

Kristen Checks In

(Saturday, August 24, 2002)

At last, the day came for Kristen to check into the hospital. Having spent the previous several months not knowing what would happen from one week to the next, it now felt kind of surreal to know the operation was only a few days away.

Although we were all having eleventh-hour jitters, it was good to know we were in the hands of world-renowned surgeons. We were also a lot better prepared than when Kristen had first been admitted four months earlier.

After Kristen checked in, she was put in a room down the hall from the nurses' station. I would be put in the room next to hers when I was admitted on Tuesday, so we could be close to each other. It was these extra considerations that meant a lot to us, and showed that the nursing staff really thought of everything.

As I'd said to my convention colleagues back in Raleigh, this was going to be a strange experience for me. The IWK staff had been through this kind of thing hundreds of times, but at 51, I would be checking into a hospital for the first time in my life—and a children's hospital at that.

As we sat in Kristen's room and the reality of my upcoming admission began to sink in, I started to feel a little panicked. Our roles were suddenly reversed, and now it was Kristen's turn to talk me through a stressful situation. At that moment, she seemed unbelievably calm and composed. I didn't realize that she was quietly dealing with her own fears as well.

KRISTEN REMEMBERS…

I remember feeling apprehensive about the surgery once I read the list of side effects that went with the cocktail of medications I would soon be taking for the rest of my life. They included both hair loss (on my head) and hair growth (everywhere else), acne, moon face, weight gain, jaundice—oh, and cancer.

Quite a list for anyone to look at. Imagine reading that as an already-anxious 15-year-old girl.

I wanted to be "normal" and to look "normal" once this whole ordeal was done. I remember thinking, "WHAT THE HELL! I just almost died and have gone through ridiculous amounts of pain and torment, and NOW I have to take a cocktail of drugs that is going to make me bald, fat, and a pizza face... GREAT!"

That day, we received an email from Bob, a friend in New Glasgow, letting us know that he'd spoken with his sister, Sue.

I had met Sue years earlier, back in university. When hanging out in the campus residence with Sully and Bob, I would often go to the nurses' residence with the boys to visit her and the other nurses she hung around with. I didn't even know that she'd become an operating-room nurse, let alone worked in the IWK, until we were close to the day of the operation.

Apparently, she had wanted to know when the operation would take place, so that she could arrange to be there. Bob assured us he would let her know the date. I really appreciated that, knowing what a comfort it would be to see a friendly face in an operating room full of masked strangers!

John Checks In

(Tuesday, August 27, 2002)

Tuesday was my day to check into the IWK. By this time, we'd gotten to know many of the staff members, and it helped me feel a little better to see their familiar faces after I'd changed from civvies into hospital garb. Most of them were aware of my lack of experience as a patient, so they did everything they could to help me feel at ease.

As promised, I was put in the room next to Kristen's. I didn't have much to unpack, just an extra set of clothes to put on when I left the hospital afterwards. (Because hospital gowns are notorious for their lack of pockets, I'd left all my valuables at home.)

At that time, every room was equipped with a TV and video player. I knew I'd be in there for at least a few days, so I'd gone to a local video store and rented some movies for my hospital stay. Hearing about my situation, they were even kind enough to just charge me a regular fee, and forgive any late fees.

The doctors ran some more tests, and then there was nothing left for us to do but wait. Because the next day was going to be a big one, our nerves had become pretty strained, so the nurses gave us both some medication—Gravol, I think—to help us feel calm.

I walked over to Kristen's room to see how she was doing. She looked so fragile. I told her that no matter how the next day turned out, I loved her with all my heart.

She said "I love you" back, and we sat for awhile, both a bit 'spacey' from the Gravol.

I knew Kristen had the same anxieties as me, but she didn't show it. I suspected that she was just looking forward to having this ordeal over with.

KRISTEN REMEMBERS...

Truthfully I was so concerned about my dad not waking up that I forgot about my own anxiety. Of course, I was worried that something would happen to me, but the greater risk was to my dad, given his age and his size. So, I didn't have much time to worry about myself.

I didn't want to show my nervousness, but inside I was anxious. For me (and I tried to keep this to myself, knowing it would sound crazy), having not been put under before, I wasn't sure whether I was going to wake up again. I just reminded myself that as long as Kristen received a healthy kidney, that was all that mattered.

I kissed her 'goodbye' and went back to my room. Thanks to the medication, I soon fell asleep.

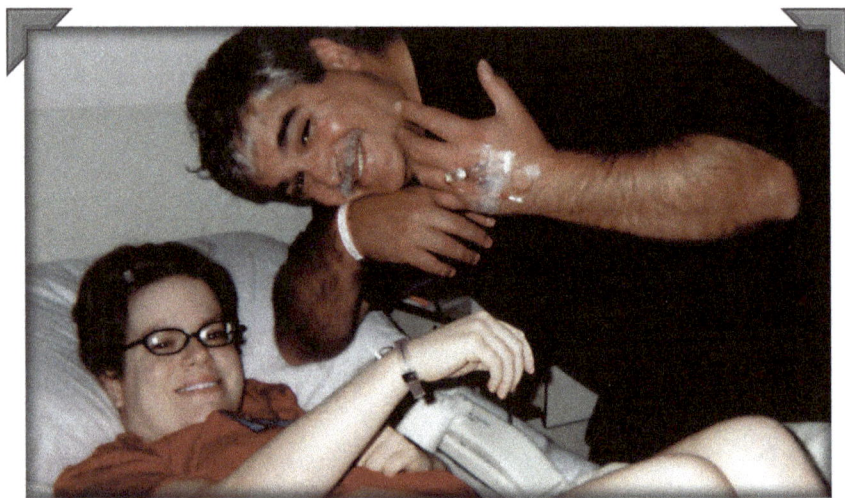

Showing off our IVs.

The Big Day

(Wednesday, August 28, 2002)

The next morning began early for me. I showered at around 4 a.m., put on a hospital gown, and waited for a nurse to come get me for the operation.

I hadn't been allowed to eat since before midnight because my stomach would have to be empty when the surgery began. Around 7 a.m., they gave me another anxiety pill. Then a nurse helped me into a wheelchair and took me down to the elevators.

When we got to the operating room floor, I met up with Kristen and Debbie. We held hands for a short while, and then—too quickly—Kristen had to go. I kissed her and told her I would see her very soon, and Debbie and I watched as she was wheeled around the corner—out of our sight, once again.

I couldn't help but think that something terrible was going to happen and this was the last time I would see her. I didn't care about myself, but death should never come to someone so young.

Soon, I was wheeled into an operating room, leaving Debbie on her own. I could only imagine what she was going through, and her anxiety at both her child *and* her husband being taken away from her.

Our lives were now in the doctors' hands, and although they were highly skilled, it was still terrifying to have no control over what would happen to us.

KRISTEN REMEMBERS…

I did have kind of an emotional breakdown when they went to put in the surgical IV. After having well over a dozen IVs at that point, my reaction to this particular one surprised even me.

The nurses said that I was probably so overcome with emotion and nerves that the size of this needle just put me over the edge. It seemed like they were coming at me with a knitting needle!

They agreed to wait awhile, and put the IV in when I was slightly more sedated and less emotional.

Over the previous weeks and months, time had seemed to drag. Now, everything was going almost too quickly. In a way, that was all right: I wanted the operation to be over, all of this drama to be behind us, and everything to be normal again. Yes, I was nervous, but I was also relieved that our 'train' was finally coming into the station.

Sue, my operating-nurse angel of mercy, was in the operating room when I was brought in. It felt good to talk to someone I knew, and just seeing her friendly face (well, her friendly eyes above her mask) immediately calmed me down.

Within minutes, the operation was underway.

The first order of business was an epidural. They had me sit on the side of the operating table, and the anesthesiologist felt my back for a good location. Unfortunately, he couldn't find a suitable spot between my vertebrae, so they decided that I would be hooked up the old-fashioned way—intravenously—to give me painkillers and fluids when I needed them.

They helped me lie down, a mask was put over my mouth and nose, and off to sleep I went. I was told later that they actually 'kill' (my term) your body for the operation. This is so you don't move while you're under, which could be disastrous in a delicate procedure like this.

Needless to say, I wasn't really 'present' for the next part, but I can give you a *very* basic overview of how it went.

I'll start with my part of the operation, where they removed my kidney.

When they're taking out your kidney, the way they have you lie down depends on which kidney they need, and how they're going to remove it. They often prefer to have you lie on your side, with your hip elevated above your head and feet—sort of like a jack-knife. It's not the most comfortable position, but it does give the surgery team the best possible access to your kidney.

You're then put under for the operation, and they run a Foley catheter into your bladder. This will help to drain your urine for the next 24 hours (after which the catheter will come out).

Because this happened back in 2002, they used a surgery technique called a *flank incision*. This involved making a six-inch cut in my right side, just below my ribs. This would allow them to pull the muscle aside so that they could reach my kidney more easily. With the flank incision, they would often have to remove the tip of one of your ribs to get to your kidney, so I was told beforehand that I could probably expect a lot of pain afterwards.

Nowadays they're more likely to use *laparoscopic* surgery. Instead of a big cut, they make some small, 'pinky'-sized incisions in your tummy: usually one in the belly button, a second cut a little to the side of that one, and a third cut a few inches above the belly button. These are the holes they use to insert the instruments and camera needed to perform the surgery.

Of course, when they actually take out the kidney, they need to do this through a bigger hole, so they also make a special cut, called a *bikini line* incision, just above your pubic bone. It's much smaller than the flank incision they had to make during my operation, and they don't have to remove part of your rib, so it's a big improvement over the older technique.

When they went in and located my kidney, they probably had to take a moment to confirm that the kidney was healthy and suitable for transplant. (Remember: up to that point, all they had to go on were CAT scans and X-rays.)

After confirming that my kidney was a 'go,' they were able to put Kristen under. At that point, they typically give the recipient a dosage of immune-suppressant drugs to help ensure that their body won't reject the new kidney. In Kristen's case, they used Simulect. This was a very effective drug, but as we later found out, it could also have some pretty scary side effects.

When both the donor and recipient are under, the surgery team can complete the transplant. To begin, they separate the donor's kidney from the surrounding tissue. Then they clamp off three important vessels coming out of the kidney: the *ureter* (which carries urine from the kidney to the bladder), the *renal artery* (which feeds blood *to* the kidney), and the *renal vein* (which carries blood *from* the kidney). Once these vessels are clamped shut, they cut the vessels, remove the kidney, and stitch and close up the incisions.

As soon as they remove the kidney, they transfer it to an open container. Then they pour crushed ice on top of the kidney to keep it cold. (This prevents cell and tissue damage from happening.)

They now have to quickly clear all the blood out of the kidney before it starts to clot. To do this, they open up the arteries and veins coming out of the kidney, and force a special solution into them. This solution usually contains a cocktail of ingredients, including blood thinners like Heparin. The solution is also very cold, which helps to bring down the internal temperature of the kidney.

When the kidney has cooled down enough, the next part of the operation can begin.

A kidney transplant is very different from, say, a heart or liver transplant. With the latter two, they take out your original organ and put the replacement in the exact same spot. But with a kidney transplant, they usually leave the original kidneys where they are (unless they *have* to remove them), and put the new kidney in a completely different spot, usually in your lower abdomen. Eventually, the original kidneys will shrivel up to the size of raisins, so you won't even notice them.

There are two reasons why a transplanted kidney is placed so low compared to where your kidneys normally sit: First, the blood vessels in your lower abdomen and pelvis are relatively easy to get to, which means less time on the operating table and fewer complications afterwards. Second, a lower kidney placement means that the ureter will have to run a much shorter distance from the new kidney to your bladder—again, this helps to reduce possible complications.

They begin by making an incision low in your abdomen, and pulling aside the muscle and protective layers. They locate and prepare the blood vessels they'll need to connect to your new kidney—usually an artery and vein that come from high up in your leg. Then they place the new kidney inside.

They connect the renal artery and renal vein running out of the kidney to the appropriate blood vessels. Then, they test the blood flow to make sure there are no leaks.

The kidney should now start to change from a grey to a pink colour, and it may even start to squirt out urine. (Fun fact: when a *deceased* kidney is transplanted, it doesn't just start working on its own. It has to be 'kick-started' by dialysis to get it going.)

Now it 's time to hook up the ureter. First, they insert a narrow tube, called a *stent*, into the end of the ureter, leaving part of the stent outside the ureter opening. Then, they make a small incision in your bladder. They stick the end of the ureter into the bladder, and, using a very fine suture, they sew the bladder shut around the end of the ureter.

(Another fun fact: The stent is *very* important because it stops the ureter from closing up after the operation; if it closes up, then urine cannot pass through to your bladder.)

After that, it's a matter of closing up the muscle layer and the outer skin, and they're done.

Of course, this is a really simple overview of a very difficult and delicate operation; in reality, it actually took about three hours from start (when I was first put under) to finish (when Kristen's incisions were finally closed up).

* * *

After what felt like a few seconds, I woke up. I don't remember very much of what happened then because the drugs had taken a pretty good hold on me. I do remember being wrapped up in a warm, comfortable blanket.

As I'd promised, the first things I asked were how Kristen was doing and what day it was. I was reassured that it was still the same day (in fact, it wasn't even noon), but anxious when I heard that Kristen's procedure was still underway.

A short while later, I was brought back to the sixth floor, and transferred to the bed in my room. Although I was pretty uncomfortable with all the tubes hanging out of me, I felt completely exhausted, and was soon fast asleep.

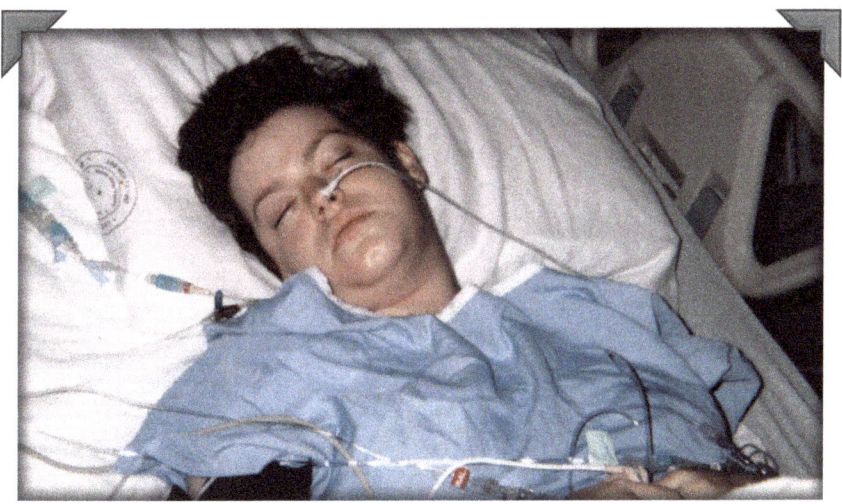

Post-op recovery

The Day After

(Thursday, August 29, 2002)

The next day, I woke up in my room, hooked up to a bunch of monitors. An IV drip ran into my arm, delivering pain medication and fluids.

I asked about Kristen and was told that her operation had been a success. She had begun peeing almost immediately after the transplant, which was a really good sign. She was now in isolation in the recovery room, and wouldn't be moved back to the sixth floor until later.

I was shown some post-op pictures of Kristen; she looked so pathetic, all swollen and bruised. She had more tubes hanging out of her than I did, but I was assured that this was normal and that they would be taken out soon.

Later, the doctors came in to check my staples. They'd used them instead of stitches because staples would heal more quickly and the resulting scar would be almost invisible.

Another piece of good news was that they hadn't needed to remove part of my rib to get to my kidney. This would mean that, although I would still experience some post-op discomfort, I would have to endure a lot less pain, not to mention a shorter healing time.

One of the nurses pointed to a button next to my bed. She said that if I needed any relief, I could press it, and pain medication would be injected right into my IV. At that point, I felt okay; in fact, it seemed like nothing worse than a pulled muscle.

KRISTEN REMEMBERS…

After the surgery, I really can't remember much other than my mom and my cousin Cheryl hanging over my bed with gowns and masks on. I wasn't in much pain YET because I was heavily sedated. My mom was so concerned for me, but I don't actually remember hearing her talk to me. Everything was muffled.

I do remember that the next day, when they transferred me from the ICU back to the sixth floor, this one particular nurse asked me to move, and I yelled at her because I was in such excruciating pain and just wanted to stay put. I felt like my insides were on fire.

* * *

While I was recuperating, a good friend of mine, Glenn MacArthur, came by. He was driving that night to Montreal on business, but stopped in to see how we were doing.

He noticed the VCR, and I told him I'd probably be up watching videos all night because I was having trouble sleeping.

Glenn was actually a bit of a night owl when it came to long-distance driving; in fact, he liked driving overnight because there was so little traffic on the road that he could make great time. Before he left, he gave me his cell phone number and asked me to call him periodically, just to make sure he hadn't fallen asleep or gone off the road.

I ended up calling him twice, and we made a game of it: before he told me where he was, I would guess his location. Both times, I was correct within a kilometre or two—not bad, considering I was both sleep-deprived and fresh out of surgery.

Of course, I knew Glenn was an excellent driver, and that the calls were mostly so he could check up on me, and make sure I was okay.

It's that kind of support that makes tough times bearable. Friends can really be a blessing.

Simulect, Take Two

(Friday, August 30, 2002)

When the doctors checked up on me the next day, they were amazed to learn that I still didn't need any painkillers. Frankly, so was I; I'd been told to expect pain like I'd never experienced before, but for the duration of my stay, I ended up having almost no discomfort at all. (In fact, I didn't have to press my pain medication button once the entire time.)

They unhooked my IV and told me that if I needed a painkiller, a prescription had been left for me at the nurses' station. (I ended up not needing that, either.)

As the effects of the drugs wore off, I did begin to feel hungry. Fortunately, I was told that I could once again eat solid food, and as much as I wanted.

Who was I to question a doctor's orders? I doubled what I ate, and if turkey was included, I tripled it! I felt alive and hopeful once again, and my appetite was certainly proof of that.

* * *

Later that day, Kristen was brought back to the sixth floor and placed in a special isolation room located right in front of the nurses' station. It was set up this way so they could keep a close eye on patients after surgery.

Kristen was then given her second dose of Simulect. The way this medication works is by suppressing your immune system so your body doesn't attack a newly transplanted organ. Of course, having a suppressed immune system also means that if you're exposed to any kind of virus or bug, you can easily catch it—so even a minor cold can make you really sick.

Because of this, only a handful of people were allowed to visit Kristen. Debbie was at the top of that list, and she had to gown and wash up thoroughly before going into Kristen's room.

Of course, this wasn't the only part of the Simulect treatment that would bring complications. In fact, the riskiest procedure still lay ahead, when Kristen was scheduled to receive her third and final shot of Simulect two weeks later.

In Recovery

(Friday, August 30, to Wednesday, September 4, 2002)

After you've had surgery, the idea is to get you moving around as quickly as possible to help speed up your recovery. By Friday, I was actually looking forward to that because I'd been on my back for a couple of days, and it was starting to get uncomfortable. That day, with the help of the nurses, I began getting out of bed and sitting in a nearby chair. (Baby steps, but at least it was a start.)

The following Monday, the doctors checked my staples and decided that they'd healed enough to be taken out. By that point, I was taking regular walks around the ward, IV pole in hand, and was able to reach the isolation room where Kristen was staying.

Seeing her on the other side of the glass, hooked up to all kinds of IVs, tubes, and monitors, was very hard to take. All I wanted to do was go in and give her a hug. Instead, we had to resort to communicating through the window, using basic sign language.

KRISTEN REMEMBERS…

Once I was feeling better, I sort of loved being in isolation because I got the peace and quiet an older sibling longs for. (I also got the TV to myself!)

It didn't even bother me that I couldn't go out and roam the halls.

Fortunately, after a few days, they were able to gown me up, put a mask on me, and let me into the isolation room. I was jittery and shaking from head to foot when I walked in, but I went over to Kristen's bed and gave her that great big hug I'd been saving.

I said I loved her and I told her everything would be fine, and we had a wonderful, but brief, visit. She was a little sore, but otherwise in good spirits, and I could see her coming back to the way she had been before all of this started.

KRISTEN REMEMBERS…

It was about a week before I could sit up without assistance, and by that point I was feeling really well. It was nice to wake up without feeling nauseous or exhausted.

However, they'd given me a steroid called Prednisone, and once it began to kick in, I was a big bundle of energy.

I had NO idea what to do with all this excess energy. I was up one night and wrote my friend Sean an email that was roughly six pages long because I just couldn't settle down.

Of course, with prednisone you also get an insatiable appetite, so I went from being severely malnourished and clinically anorexic to having an appetite like that of a sumo wrestler.

The doctors told us that Kristen would remain in isolation for at least the rest of September. Still, they said that overall, her recovery was remarkable.

* * *

Two days later, I was ready to leave the hospital. It had only been nine days since I was admitted, and I was told it was one of the quickest releases in recent memory.

Although I was happy to be going home to recuperate, it meant that I wouldn't be able to visit Kristen until I was stronger.

Before I was released from the hospital, we went to Kristen's room, and I waved good-bye to her through the window. A few minutes later, I was back in the 'real' world, sitting in our car as Debbie drove me home.

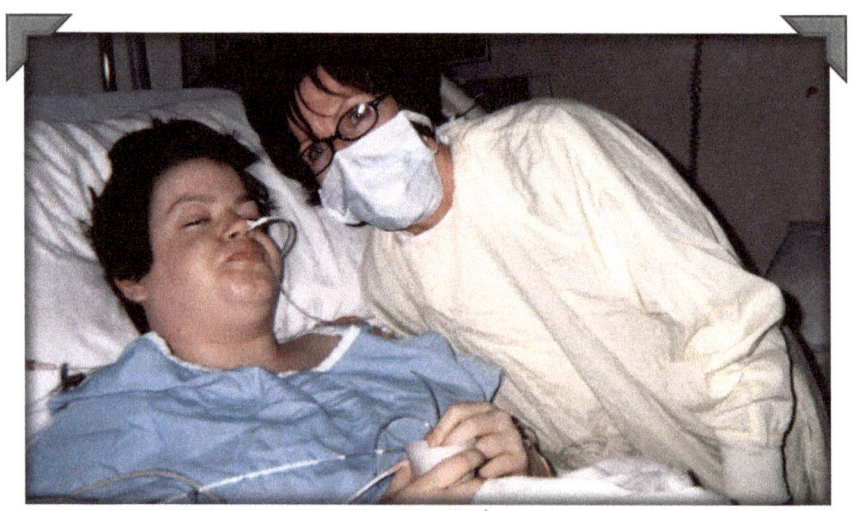

Debbie and Kristen, post-op.

Stents, Staples, and the Great Outdoors

(Friday, September 13, to Sunday, September 15, 2002)

About two weeks after the operation, Kristen had a procedure to remove her stent and staples. After the operation, they phoned us to let us know that everything had gone well. Debbie and I drove to the hospital, and waited outside the recovery room. Once again, they had to avoid exposing her to any outside germs, so they were limiting the number of visitors. We decided that Debbie would see Kristen first.

Debbie told me afterwards that by the time Kristen came back to the room, she was almost completely recovered from surgery. She was also really hungry because she hadn't been able to eat anything since midnight, and it was now 3 in the afternoon.

Two very good signs.

* * *

That weekend, the doctors told Kristen she could go outside for a couple of hours, as long as she was careful not to overtax her immune system.

KRISTEN REMEMBERS:

Two weeks post-transplant, it was unheard of by the nurses that the doctors would clear someone to be off isolation and go outside. Of course, they carefully considered everything: the state of the floor (were there any flu cases, and so on), and whether my levels were stable and I was strong enough.

That day, Kristen put on a mask for protection, and we took her out to the play-garden.

KRISTEN REMEMBERS:

I needed to wear a mask for the first month or so post-transplant and whenever I had to leave the hospital.

I ended up needing to use the mask for roughly a year after that, whenever I had to come into the hospital for lab work. Germs are rampant in a hospital, and I was in NO condition to get sick where my kidney was brand new and my immune system was so fragile.

Once Kristen was outside, she was able to take the mask off. It was wonderful to see her enjoy the fresh air, after being stuck inside for so long. We swung on the swings, walked around the play-garden, and enjoyed time as a family.

Soon it began to rain, so we decided to head back in. But Kristen stopped us; she wanted to stay outside because she enjoyed feeling the rain on her face. It's funny how something so ordinary, that many of us take for granted, can bring so much joy to someone who hasn't experienced it for awhile.

A little later, Debbie went to pick up Allison, who had been at a sleepover the previous night, and brought her back so she could join us in the play-garden.

When we returned to the sixth floor, we were told that Kristen would be able to have day passes after her third dose of Simulect. We were excited that it would be her final treatment, but also very nervous about possible side effects.

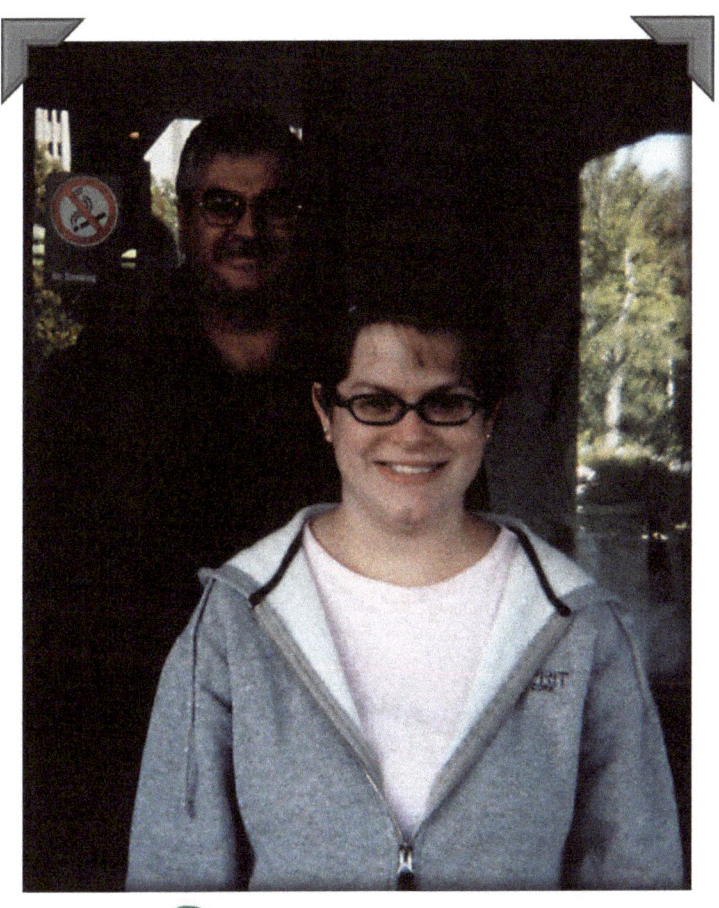

Finally-getting some fresh air!

Third Time Lucky?

(Wednesday, September 18, 2002)

Finally, the day arrived for Kristen to receive her last dose of Simulect. We were told that kids usually had a reaction to it at some point during the treatment. Apparently, the first dosage never caused a reaction, the second one occasionally, and the third one—almost always.

The doctors assured us that if Kristen had a reaction, it would be short-lived. But they warned us that it could still be frightening: if it happened, her breathing passage would swell up, and she would feel like she was choking.

Because the symptoms would appear as soon as she received the shot, the doctors and nurses were prepared to respond immediately. Poor Debbie had to leave the room because she couldn't bear to see anything happen.

We all held our breath as they administered the third shot...

...and...

...Nothing!

There was no reaction.

After all our worrying, we'd been stressed out for no reason. Instead, it ended up being a pretty boring experience (in the best sense of the word). On top of that, now that the Simulect treatment was finally over, they were able to take out Kristen's IV because it was no longer necessary.

We decided to celebrate by going outside to the play-garden and enjoying the beautiful day.

PART VI

Different Lives

Checked Out!

(Monday, September 23, to Friday, September 27, 2002)

The following Monday, we received some very good news: the results of Kristen's latest biopsy had come in, and there were no signs that her body was rejecting the new kidney. This meant her anti-rejection meds were working (although with a few side effects).

KRISTEN REMEMBERS...
Considering all the possible side effects I could have experienced, I ended up being pretty lucky.

I suffered from hair growth, acne, moon face, and a bit of weight gain, but that was it—and the acne was localized to my back and chest instead of my face, so I really couldn't complain too much.

On top of that, Kristen's recovery had been a record-breaker, as she'd only needed to stay in post-op isolation for two weeks. The usual time was a month.

There was still a problem with her blood pressure being too high, so just to be safe, the doctors decided to keep her under observation for a few extra days.

* * *

That Friday, I sent out an email to everyone on our mailing list to let them know the big news: after 6 months, 2 days, 4 hours, and 31 minutes (okay, give or take that last part), Kristen had finally been released from the hospital! She was coming home for good.

The night before, she'd been so excited that she couldn't sleep. Needless to say, so were we. Everyone was anxious to have her back home again.

Unfortunately, our happiness was overshadowed by a dark reality. Of course, we were grateful that Kristen was doing well and that we could finally take her home. But we were also leaving folks behind, many of whom were still in limbo—and in some cases, waiting for a miracle. We also knew that some of them might not be visited by that miracle before their time ran out. When you become friends with people who are going through this, their suffering can feel as devastating as if it's your own—and it haunts you for a long time afterward.

At the same time, we were also seeing the end of many relationships we had forged with people who worked at the hospital. These were wonderful, caring individuals who had helped us, not just through some of our most difficult and frightening moments, but also through the day-to-day business of surviving and coping.

Of course, Kristen would still have follow-up visits—scheduled blood tests and biopsies would bring us back—so we would see some of them again. But many of those friendly faces that we had come to look forward to each day would now disappear from our lives forever.

All of these relationships with so many inspirational people—both patients and staff—had profoundly affected us. We weren't the same family that had walked into the hospital six months earlier; whatever challenges the future held, we would now take them on with greater strength and confidence, and (I think) more wisdom. One thing that this experience had taught us was how important it is to prepare for any medical situation with as much knowledge as possible.

KRISTEN REMEMBERS…

I am so tainted by this whole experience that any doctor I have knows that I will drill them with questions to ensure that I am getting the best care.

Being your own advocate is so important, and my only hope from this book is that people understand that you must ask questions and be prepared to take action when it comes to your family's health and well-being. People must understand that although doctors are generally very skilled and knowledgeable, at the end of the day, they are still human and capable of making mistakes. And sometimes, these mistakes can be catastrophic.

Post-op Biopsies

(Monday, November 25, to Wednesday, November 27, 2002)

On a chilly Monday in late November, Kristen checked in overnight at the IWK hospital for her scheduled three-month biopsy. The next day, they performed the procedure, without a hitch.

KRISTEN REMEMBERS…

With a kidney transplant, they usually schedule biopsies for one month, three months, six months, and a year afterward. I eventually ended up needing an extra one at nine months because my creatinine and urea levels were slightly elevated.

We got the lab results back on Wednesday. The doctors found that Kristen had a spillover of sugar in her urine, which wasn't too serious, but they also found *E. coli*, which could be a problem. The bacteria was in her bladder, so they gave her antibiotics to make sure it didn't travel north (or in her case, sideways) into her new kidney.

We suspected she might have picked up the infection between the previous Tuesday (her last blood-and-urine test day) and Sunday, when she began her new round of tests. Of course, it was difficult to say for sure; Kristen was so immune-suppressed from the anti-rejection drugs that she could have picked it up anywhere.

Meanwhile, my incision was healing pretty well. Thanks to a wooden cane that a buddy of mine, Cliff Boudreau, had made for me, I even managed to hobble up the stairs to the press box for the opening day of football season at Saint Mary's. (My old friend Rusty had volunteered to fill in as an announcer on any games that I was unable to attend, but as it turned out, I didn't miss any.)

Another pleasant surprise: the doctors didn't expect me to be able to play golf until the following season, but I confounded them by going out six weeks after the operation, in mid-October. In fact, I managed six trips to the greens that fall before they closed the course on us!

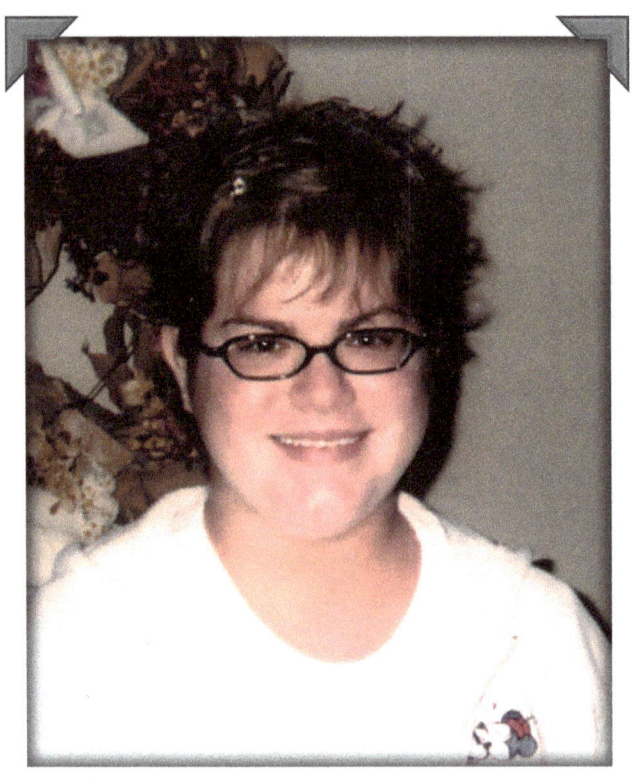

Three months post-op — feeling like a normal teen!

Back to School

(October 2002 to June 2005)

Kristen started her Grade 10 classes in October of that year. Because she'd only been out of the hospital for about a month and was still recovering, they decided that she would only attend classes for half of each day. Still, everyone was amazed at how much she had changed since the spring.

KRISTEN REMEMBERS...

All of my stars realigned. I had really awesome grades, some really great relationships, and my life was on track. I finally felt like a normal teenager—I mean, sure, my life had changed and sure, I had to take medications around the clock, but I was now a teenager living my life and not worrying about losing my life!

Even though she wasn't able to attend full time, she made up for that with her enthusiasm and positive attitude. Her teachers noticed that she was doing a lot more work and of much better quality. This was a huge vindication for Kristen: she could now show them that she'd been capable of doing the work all along, and would easily have completed Grade 9 had it not been for her kidney disease.

Kristen met regularly with her teachers to discuss her medical and academic progress. They also helped her figure out how to catch up given the fact that she'd started late, missing half of the semester. One solution they devised was to develop exams based only on what Kristen had actually been in class for.

KRISTEN REMEMBERS...

My entire school experience was now so much better: my teachers were empathetic instead of being critical, and they made it a point to help me succeed rather than judge me for failing. I wasn't a failure and I wasn't slow; I just needed a little bit of help and a little bit of understanding rather than being branded as a lazy, ignorant student.

Everyone was so pleased to have the real Kristen back, and she worked hard to catch up with the class, while also enjoying time with her friends. Through the follow-up biopsies, and despite the side effects from the *thirteen* different medications she was now on, Kristen took on every challenge she encountered, both in school and in her personal life. In June 2005, she received her high school diploma.

KRISTEN REMEMBERS…

I had one complication three years after the transplant. I was 18, and it happened just after senior prom. Dr. Acott reaffirmed that it wasn't even a rejection; it was just a blip, but enough of a blip that they didn't want to take any chances.

I was given a drug called Solu-Medrol, which contains a very concentrated dose of prednisone. They used pulse therapy, which meant that they gave me the drug over the course of a week and a bit, starting at high volumes, and eventually reducing it to pills once the dosage was more manageable.

I was so UPSET when I had this rejection because I had just lost over 60 pounds for prom and was feeling really good about myself, and then all of a sudden I had a setback. Still, I was determined to keep the weight off, and I did—despite my prednisone-induced food cravings rearing their ugly heads.

University

(September 2005 to May 2014)

For a long time, Kristen had thought about becoming a teacher. By the time she finished high school, she was fluent in French, and so she set her sights on teaching French to elementary students.

With Kristen's post-op care foremost in our minds, Debbie and I hoped that Kristen would earn her degree at St. Mary's University. The campus was only a ten-minute drive from our home, and it was just a few minutes' walk from several major hospitals, including the IWK. Unfortunately, when we looked into it, we learned that the school no longer had an education program.

In the 1990s, the provincial government had cut back on funding to all of the universities, and one of the targeted programs was teacher education. This led to consolidation, and St. Mary's was one of the universities forced to shut down their education program. Although Kristen could earn her arts degree at St. Mary's, she would have to earn her Bachelor of Education degree somewhere else.

As it turned out, this was okay with Kristen, because she actually wanted to earn her teaching degree at St. Francis Xavier University (or St. F.X., as the students call it).

Debbie and I both knew that St. F.X. was an excellent school, with an exceptional teaching program. What concerned us, though, was that the St. F.X. campus was located in Antigonish, a town about two hours' drive from Halifax.

This meant that if Kristen needed hospital care, adding those two hours of travelling time to the equation—possibly on winter roads and at high speeds—could easily turn a small complication into a life-threatening crisis.

Of course, because Kristen hadn't even begun her undergraduate studies, we wouldn't be crossing that bridge for some time, but as her parents, Debbie and I had to think about these things.

In September 2005, Kristen enrolled in the Arts undergraduate program at St. Mary's.

*   *   *

Although Kristen did well in her studies, her time at St. Mary's was sometimes complicated by health issues. At one point, she developed mononucleosis, which meant that she had to withdraw for an entire semester. Although she was very disappointed, she had little choice; it made her feel tired all the time and she couldn't concentrate on her studies.

In spite of this setback, the beginning of the next semester saw her back at school, and she worked hard to earn her degree over the following years. She graduated with a Bachelor of Arts, majoring in French, in May 2012.

KRISTEN REMEMBERS…
It took so long because I had to switch to part-time enrolment, taking only two to three courses each year.

Just as when she'd finished high school, we were all so proud of her. This time, she'd earned a university degree while also dealing with the side effects from her medications and her other health issues, on top of all the usual challenges a student has to face. She'd proven that she could handle it, which made us feel more comfortable about her next step.

*   *   *

Kristen's dream finally came true when, in September 2012, she enrolled in the Education program at St. Francis Xavier. It would be the first time she was really away from home, but her condition was stable enough—and she was mature enough—that we felt, well, *okay* about her being so far away from us. We also learned that if any complications arose, there were hospitals in Antigonish that could provide the care she needed, so she wouldn't have to travel to Halifax.

We also weren't afraid that she would become careless about her meds, which is often a problem with students who have had transplants. Since day one, Kristen had confronted the disease with a lot of maturity and responsibility; she understood that taking her anti-rejection medication regularly, and avoiding drugs and alcohol, were necessary to keep her healthy.

Sadly, a lot of young people who have received transplants, upon feeling better, don't continue with their meds and then wind up with a rejected kidney or other serious problems. Being both at university and away from home for the first time, it's easy to lose your sense of balance. Seeing everyone else drinking and partying, you can quickly become convinced that you're just as indestructible. Too late, you discover that you're not.

* * *

Although we never worried about Kristen being irresponsible, it didn't mean that we never worried. In fact, I vividly remember one crisp fall day in November 2013, when Kristen was in her final year at St. F.X. She was doing her school practicum, so she was living at home at the time.

KRISTEN REMEMBERS…

I attended St. F.X., but we had the option to do our practice teaching at a school closer to home. So I did two months of study at St. F.X. for each term and two months of practicums at a local elementary school.

She had just left for the school where she was teaching as part of a French immersion program.

"Bye, Daddy, see you after school!" she said, rushing out the door. She was excited to see her students for the second day.

I had just finished emptying the dishwasher, and was standing in the kitchen, eating a bowl of cereal. Then, out of the blue, I suddenly imagined Kristen rushing home, and banging on the door to get in. I saw myself open the door to find her standing there with blood streaming out of her nose, screaming that something was wrong.

Even though this was all in my head, it seemed so vivid. Over the years, I've managed to shelve those terrible thoughts and fears in the back of my mind, but every once in a while, they come racing back: a thousand different nightmares that I pray we will never have to experience.

Fortunately, on that particular day, my imagination was overactive, just like it had been so many times before. Kristen came home after work, completely fine, with only stories of her day at school—and nothing else.

Although nothing had gone wrong that day, as any parent knows, your mind will create all kinds of worst-case scenarios on its own. I suppose it does this so you'll be prepared if and when any of these terrible things actually happen. I guess that's a good thing, but it sure can add some years onto your life.

A New Journey

Spring and Fall of 2014

In the spring of 2014, Kristen graduated from St. F.X., earning her degree in Education. She was older than most of her fellow grads, but she had also been an older-than-usual entrant to the program. I think that her maturity helped her keep her priorities straight, and her past experience at St. Mary's had taught her to balance her health with her studies. Now, after all the challenges she'd taken on and won over the previous 12 years, she could proudly wear the special 'X' ring, one of the most recognized grad rings around the world.

Like many of her fellow grads, Kristen was now concentrating on finding work. Although teaching jobs were scarce in Halifax, Kristen did have two things going for her: she'd majored in French for her undergraduate degree at St. Mary's, and there was a shortage of French immersion teachers in Halifax.

With so many years of formal education behind her, Kristen couldn't wait to start helping young students on their own journeys. However, getting into any system can take time, and Kristen was told she wouldn't be able to start teaching until September. In the meantime, she spent the summer getting as many shifts as she could at a local big box store.

Later that summer, she was thrilled to find out that one of the schools where she'd taught for her practicum had asked that she come back. They needed someone to fill in for a deferred leave, and the principal offered her the position.

In the fall of 2014, Kristen started her first job as a teacher.

John: The Fear Never Leaves

Kristen has always been an advocate for her health, and because of her experience, she knows all the symptoms to look out for. Unfortunately, when she feels anxious, those symptoms can become amplified.

When she phones me with a problem, I never let on that I'm worried, because I want her to keep me up to date on her health. I'd rather stay in the loop and deal with the occasional scare—especially if the alternative is to be kept in the dark, and always wondering if she's okay.

I also like to think I can be of some help. Once she hears my calming voice (yes, I know: ironic), she seems to settle down, and soon realizes that whatever is wrong has nothing to do with her kidney. She's almost never had symptoms that led to a hospital visit, and she's never had a really serious setback. God forbid that she ever does—you might as well dig a second hole for me!

Actually, it's often a wait-and-see situation for both of us. I'm not a doctor, so I have to see where each call takes us. Every time, it's sort of like running a course of hurdles, and my heart takes a while to settle down afterwards. Fortunately, I haven't lost any sleep lately, and her recent calls aren't as dramatic as in the early days, when she was away at university.

Although I start each call assuming the worst, by the end of the conversation, I'm letting out a huge sigh of relief and giving a little prayer of thanks.

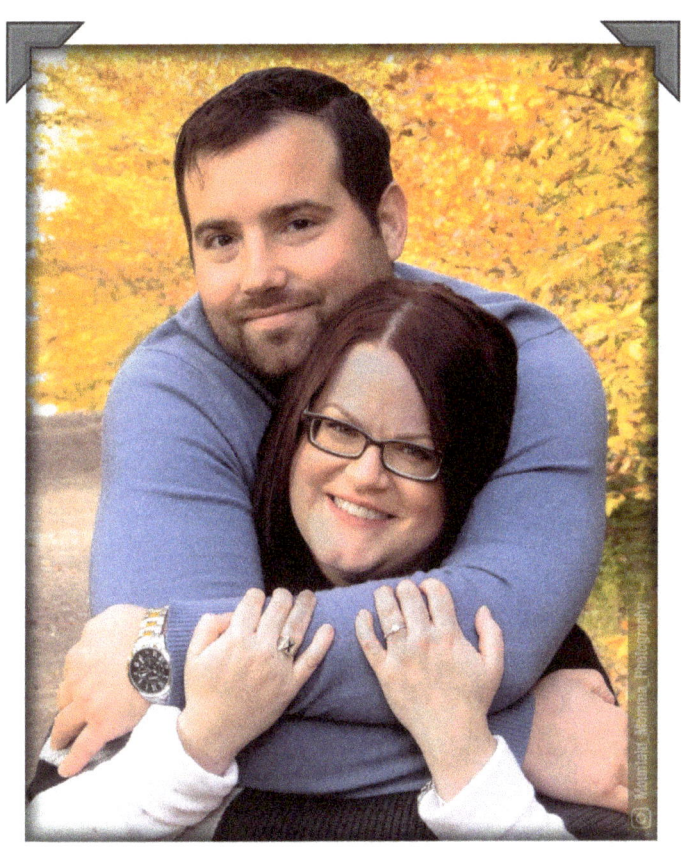

The happy couple!

Kristen: Looking Forward

Seventeen years ago, I endured a series of trials and tribulations that started me on the road to who I am today. I am an advocate for myself in every way. I didn't let all those events define what I would be capable of later in life.

Yes, it sucks that I'll be "handicapped" by this disease, and all that it entails, for the remainder of my life; but there are people in far worse shape than me, and I do everything I can to ensure that I'm not caught off guard like I was in 2002. I take very good care of my kidney and I do everything possible to maintain its health. Still, there is only so much that's under my control. All I can do is take preventive measures to keep it alive and strong for as long as possible.

When I was 15, I asked if I would be able to have children someday. Now that I'm 32 and married, I understand that the answer is complicated. Some things that people take for granted, such as being able to have children, will not involve a normal process for me, and I am prepared to deal with that.

Living with a kidney transplant is something that comes with risks and rewards. The risks are that I could lose the kidney suddenly or develop cancer from the medications that I am taking, but the reward is that I get to live a relatively normal life, free from a machine. To me, the risks are absolutely worth it.

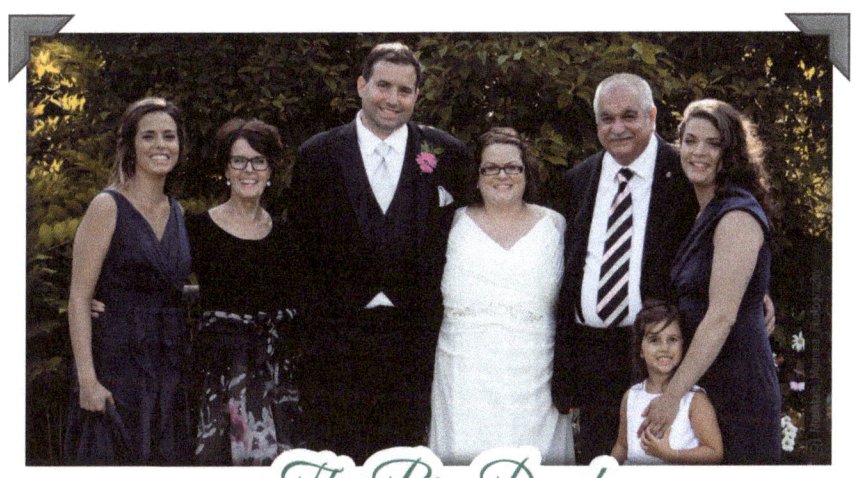

The Big Day!
(l to r) Danielle, Debbie, Rodney, Kristen, John, Aubrey, and Allison

Afterword

Thank you for reading our story.

It sat in the back of my mind for a very long time, and I am very excited to finally see it published.

I'll admit that, although it's been an emotionally rewarding experience, it's also been a difficult one. Writing about the events of that year often meant reliving them, and those moments were sometimes very painful.

For me, this process has been a sobering reminder of how close I came to losing my daughter. It has also reminded me of how lucky I have been to see her grow up, and into such an amazing person. After taking on so many incredible challenges, she has focused on following her childhood dreams and is now doing what she's always wanted to do. She's an inspiration to me, to her students, and to anyone who is lucky enough to know her.

In the 17 years since that terrible summer, our physical scars have long since healed. But a solid core of memories still remain. We learned some hard lessons, and they have affected the way we approach new doctors and our health in general. But we also have memories of some amazing people who we met during that time. Many of them we haven't seen or spoken to in years; others are no longer with us. Nevertheless, they all touched our lives in some way, and many of them showed grace and dignity in the face of circumstances that would break other people.

With that in mind, I want to leave you with a final thought:

Most doctors do their best to keep their patients healthy—not an easy thing to do these days. As patients, our job is to help them, by watching our diet, trying to be more active, making better life choices, and paying attention when our bodies warn us of problems. By working together with our doctors, we can often solve many problems before they become serious.

But some diseases don't follow the same rules that we do. They may be with us at birth, hiding in our genes, like congenital heart disease or cancer. Or, they may show up later in life but still attack us quietly on the inside, like kidney disease.

At the beginning of this story, I mentioned that kidney disease is called the 'silent killer.' That's because you don't show any symptoms until it's very advanced. Fortunately, modern medicine can help your doctor detect chronic kidney disease early on. This means you can change your lifestyle to help slow the progression of the disease before it's too late.

If a creatinine test isn't already part of your regular blood work, ask your doctor to include it. Although once a year should be adequate, you may need to have the test more often if you're at risk for certain health problems, like heart disease, high blood pressure, or if there's a history of kidney disease in your family.

I also recommend that you go online and find out how to keep your kidneys healthy and happy; you may be surprised to learn how closely related the health of your kidneys is to your general health.

One more thing: if your kidneys are healthy, I would ask you to think about registering as a donor. Your gift could be a lifeline to someone who is suffering from this terrible disease, and a chance for them to return to living a normal, productive life. In Kristen's case, I've always been thankful that I was able to provide that second chance.

All the best,
John C. Bishop

CPSIA information can be obtained
at www.ICGtesting.com
Printed in the USA
BVHW052321080122
625755BV00004BB/29